Emerging Frontiers in the Drug Formulation Design

Edited by Rahul Shukla
and Shubhini A. Saraf

Published in London, United Kingdom

Emerging Frontiers in the Drug Formulation Design
http://dx.doi.org/10.5772/intechopen.1004679
Edited by Rahul Shukla and Shubhini A. Saraf

Contributors
Abdur Mirajkar, Angeliki Siamidi, Bhuvanesh Yathavan, Dongwei Guo, Go Kimura, Hans Leuenberger, Ioanna Papoutsi, Jiayi Chen, Jingjun Huang, Mansi Singh, Maria Gazouli, Marilena Vlachou, Michael Levin, Natassa Pippa, Nefeli Lagopati, Ofer Aqua, Pranav Y. Dave, Rahul Shukla, Rahul Shukla, Shubhini A. Saraf, Stephan Schmidt, Vaibhavi Patel, Zhifeng Zhao

First published in London, United Kingdom, 2025 by IntechOpen
IntechOpen is the global imprint of INTECHOPEN LIMITED, registered in England and Wales, registration number: 11086078, 167-169 Great Portland Street, London, W1W 5PF, United Kingdom

For EU product safety concerns: IN TECH d.o.o., Prolaz Marije Krucifikse Kozulić 3, 51000 Rijeka, Croatia, info@intechopen.com or visit our website at intechopen.com.

British Library Cataloguing-in-Publication Data
A catalogue record for this book is available from the British Library

Emerging Frontiers in the Drug Formulation Design
Edited by Rahul Shukla and Shubhini A. Saraf
p. cm.

This title is part of the Pharmaceutical Science Book Series, Volume 13
Topic: Drug Discovery and Delivery
Series Editor: Rosario Pignatello
Topic Editor: Marilena Vlachou

Print ISBN 978-1-83634-245-8
Online ISBN 978-1-83634-244-1
eBook (PDF) ISBN 978-1-83634-246-5
ISSN 3033-3318

If disposing of this product, please recycle the paper responsibly.

IntechOpen Book Series
Pharmaceutical Science
Volume 13

Aims and Scope of the Series

Pharmaceutical science focuses on the design, synthesis, formulation, targeting, distribution, safety, and efficacy of active compounds as potential therapeutics. It is a large interdisciplinary discipline that aims to integrate the basic principles of physical and organic chemistry, biochemistry, biology, and engineering to discover, develop, and characterize active compounds and to optimize the formulation and delivery of drugs in the body for offering new and improved safe and efficacious therapies against human diseases. The research areas covered by the pharmaceutical sciences range from medicinal chemistry and pharmaceutical technology to pharmacology and toxicology, which represent the preliminary phases of drug development. Medicinal chemistry involves the design and synthesis of pharmaceuticals as well as the isolation of active agents from natural sources. Computer-aided strategies are increasingly involved in this drug discovery process. Pharmaceutics is a multidisciplinary science that examines the relationships between drug formulation, delivery, distribution, and clinical outcomes. Modern clinical approaches are increasingly relying on controlled release strategies and drug delivery and targeting systems, including nanotechnological platforms (nanomedicine). Pharmacology is the science of drug action in biological systems. Pharmacologists also make drugs as tools to explore aspects of cell and tissue functions. Toxicology is the study of the adverse effects of active agents on living organisms and the ecosystem, including the prevention and amelioration of such adverse effects. This book series includes volumes on Drug Discovery, Delivery, and Pharmacology. Their overall aim is to present the latest research in the whole path of drug discovery and development from different points of view of this multidisciplinary and dynamic field.

Meet the Series Editor

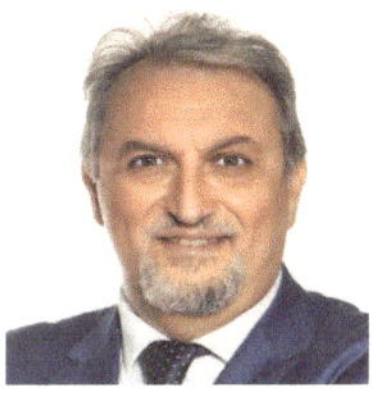

Prof. Rosario Pignatello is a Full Professor of Pharmaceutical Technology and Legislation at the University of Catania, Italy. He is the Director of the Department of Drug and Health Sciences. He has nearly 30 years of experience in the research and development of innovative formulations for the controlled release and targeting of bioactive molecules, through chemical approaches as well as nanotechnological carriers, aimed at treating different disorders. Prof. Pignatello has coauthored about 180 papers and edited a series of textbooks on biomaterials and their application in medicine. The main areas of his research are polymeric and lipid-based micro- and nanoparticles as modified drug delivery systems; vesicular nanocarriers (liposomes, micelles); lipophilic prodrugs and conjugates; synthesis and evaluation of new polymeric biomaterials for drug delivery and tissue regeneration. In particular, Prof. Pignatello works actively in the field of ocular drug delivery, leading the Research Centre for Ocular Nanotechnology, within the NANOMED Centre (Centre for Nanomedicine and Pharmaceutical Nanotechnology) at the University of Catania.

Meet the Volume Editors

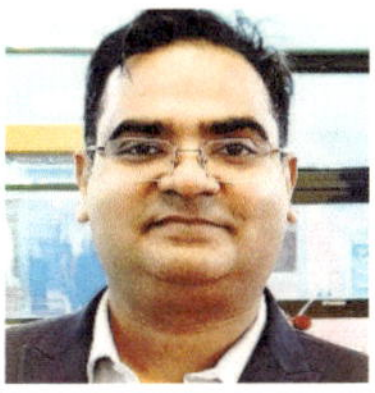

Dr. Rahul Shukla is currently working as an Assistant Professor in the Department of Pharmaceutics at NIPER Raebareli, Lucknow, an Institute of National Importance under the Ministry of Chemicals and Fertilizers, Government of India. He is listed in the Top 2% Scientists on the Stanford List in Pharmaceutical Sciences worldwide. He was awarded the SERB International Research Experience (SIRE) Fellowship for the year 2022-2023 at the School of Pharmacy and Biomedical Sciences, University of Central Lancashire, United Kingdom. Dr. Shukla has experience as a Research Scientist at Dr. Reddy's Laboratories, India, and as a D.S. Kothari Post-Doctoral Fellow at UIPS, Panjab University, India. He has over ten years of research and academic experience. He has published over 120 papers in international peer-reviewed journals and 50 book chapters. He filed 11 patents and 1 copyright. He is an editor for over 7 books published by Elsevier, Springer Nature, and IntechOpen Publishers. His publications include journals such as the *Journal of Controlled Release, Molecular Pharmaceutics, International Journal of Pharmaceutics, Expert Opinion, Journal of Drug Targeting, Colloids Surface A & B, Biomaterial Advances, Molecular Neurobiology*, and *RSC Advances,* among others. Dr. Shukla has received funding for his research from DST SERB, AYUSH, and UPCST. Dr. Shukla is a member of the Institutional Animal Ethics Committee and the Institution's Innovation Committee. He is also a member of the editorial board of the Scientific Reports journal.

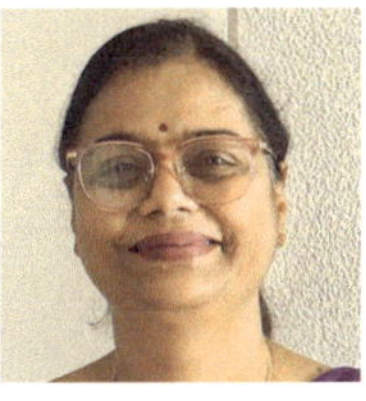

Prof. Shubhini A. Saraf currently serves as the Director of the National Institute of Pharmaceutical Education and Research (NIPER), Raebareli, India. Prior to this, she was a Professor in the Department of Pharmaceutical Sciences and Director (R&D) at Babasaheb Bhimrao Ambedkar University (A Central University), Lucknow. Prof. Shubhini's academic journey began forty years ago at the Department of Pharmaceutical Sciences, Dr. Harisingh Gour University, Sagar, India, where she completed her B. Pharm, M. Pharm, and Ph.D. in Pharmaceutical Sciences. With over 28 years of teaching and research experience, she has made significant contributions to the field. Her research interests include lipid nanoparticles, nanotechnology through material science research, principles of green nanotechnology, drug targeting approaches, and various techniques of in vitro and in vivo evaluation, such as drug bio-distribution, as well as molecular pharmaceutics and the regulation of cellular markers as indicators of health status. Her work has had a profound impact on the field. She is also actively involved in healthcare technology policy interventions. Prof. Shubhini has an impressive publication record, with more than 180 papers and 22 book chapters to her credit, and is a respected figure in the pharmacy profession.

Contents

Preface

The continuous therapeutic advancement in pharmaceutical science has led to the exploration of novel delivery systems and dosage forms. Drug formulation design is pivotal in efficient targeting and safer drug delivery methods. Innovative drug delivery systems address the demand for improved bioavailability, controlled drug release, minimized off-target effects, precise delivery, and reduced toxicity. The book "Emerging Frontiers in the Drug Formulation Design" has been edited to provide a detailed discussion on the landscape of drug formulation design.

The book is designed by subject experts, with each chapter explaining the most significant breakthroughs in modern drug formulation technologies. Delivery systems, such as liposomes, nanocrystals, and other nano-delivery systems, along with their smart features in targeted accumulation and release, are highlighted. Furthermore, the role of these nano-delivery systems in modifying bioavailability and the therapeutic fate of the drug is explained. The advanced therapeutic administration concepts of microneedles and stimuli-responsive systems are also discussed. Apart from delivery systems, optimization and drug release mechanisms are detailed, offering a deeper understanding of the behaviors of drug delivery systems and their anticipated therapeutic outcomes. Upon exploring the content of this book, researchers and students will gain insights into emerging technologies and revolutionary designs for improving patient compliance and enhancing the therapeutic potential of drugs.

Dr. Rahul Shukla
Department of Pharmaceutics,
National Institute of Pharmaceutical Education and Research-Raebareli,
Lucknow, India

Prof. Shubhini A. Saraf
Director,
National Institute of Pharmaceutical Education and Research-Raebareli,
Lucknow, India

Section 1

Nanoengineering in Drug Delivery

Chapter 1

Introductory Chapter: Redefining the Therapeutic Landscape of the Smart Drug Delivery System

Rahul Shukla and Shubhini A. Saraf

1. Introduction

The evaluation of therapeutic strategies made a notable advancement in the segment of drug delivery. The conventional dosage form has major drawbacks like poor bioavailability and nonspecific drug distribution leading to suboptimal therapeutic concentration at the site of action and repeated dosing results in exposure to systemic toxicity, non-compliance, repeated dosing, development of resistance, etc. [1]. These challenges developed an interest in the innovative approach that improves therapeutic efficacy through controlled and targeted delivery. The smart drug delivery strategy aims to deliver the therapeutic moieties to specific sites, to have control over the drug release, and to modify the physiochemical and pharmacodynamic properties of drugs [2]. Smart drug delivery is a group of concepts with a primary focus on stimuli-responsive systems, nanocarrier delivery systems, and targeted delivery systems [3]. The stimuli-responsive delivery system offers precise drug release at the site based on various external and internal stimuli such as pH, temperature, magnetic field, and enzyme activity [4]. The concept of targeted delivery or targeted distribution is majorly based on the delivery system characteristics and the expression of unique receptors or overexpression of specific receptors under particular disease conditions or at the organ site [5, 6]. Extensive research has also been conducted on nanoparticles and nanoparticles for targeted delivery or targeted release systems [7]. The unique size of the carrier will enhance the bioavailability of the therapeutic agents [8] and the addition of the concept of targeted delivery and a stimuli-responsive delivery system is anticipated to meet the current need in the management of diseases like cancer, neurological disorders, pain management, infectious diseases, and other chronic diseases [9, 10].

2. Materials and technologies in smart drug delivery

To validate the hypothesis of a smart drug delivery system, it is essential to synthesize a novel material that can meet the predetermined specifications required for the delivery system. A few examples of specific materials available for the designing of nanomaterials are different types of phospholipids (egg/soybean phosphatidylcholine, phosphatidylserine, phosphatidylglycerol, etc.) for liposomes [11]; polymers like polyamidoamine, polypropyleneimine for dendrimer [12]; polylactic acid, polycaprolactone, chitosan, dextran, etc., for polymeric nanoparticles [13]; amphiphilic polymers [poly(ethylene oxide)-b-poly(propylene oxide), poly(ethylene glycol)-grafted-poly (lactic acid), etc.] for micelles [14]. As these materials are administered systemically, they essentially degrade in the system to form non-toxic byproduct that reflects on the lower risk of accumulation and toxicity [15]. Apart from the materials required for the preparation of nanocarriers, materials capable of showing a response to stimuli have also been developed [16]. Polyphosphazene, pluronic-127 and F68, poly(N-isopropyl acrylamide) (PNIPAAM), and poly(oligo ethylene glycol methacrylate) (POEGMA) are some examples of thermosensitive polymers utilized in the development of thermal responsive drug delivery system [17]. Chemical bonds like imine bonds, amide bonds, hydrazone bones, and ester bonds are commonly present in pH-responsive polymers, which show greater drug release in acidic pH than in comparison to the normal physiological pH (7.4) [18]. Enzyme-responsive delivery systems are developed where the drug release is based on enzymes like lipase, hyaluronidase, protease, etc., which assist in the targeted release in bacterial infection conditions [19]. Further, researchers have developed a dual-functional delivery system that can achieve targeted distribution with the assistance of a functional group on the surface and targeted release with the assistance of the stimuli-responsive carrier material [20]. With the aid of a controlled release delivery system, control over drug release kinetics includes prolonged therapeutic effects, reduced dosing frequency, and fewer plasma level fluctuations have been achieved [21]. With the adaptation of these technologies, various nano-delivery systems have been developed for the management of various diseases (**Table 1** and **Figure 1**).

Sr. no.	Delivery system	Category	Drug	Outcome	Reference
1	Injectable liposomes	Pain management	Opiorphin	Reduced rapid elimination and show prolonged pain killing effect	[22]
2	Solid lipid nanoparticles	Pain management	Nalbuphine	Safe and effective in producing an analgesic effect in the brain	[23]
3	Copper nanoparticles	Infection	Atovaquone	Prophylactic effects of copper nanoparticles against chronic toxoplasmosis	[24]
4	Micelles	Infection	Efavirenz	Efficiently targeted the brain to treat HIV infection in the brain	[25]
5	Silica nanoparticles	Cancer	Doxorubicin	Excellent photothermal conversion capability and enhanced anti-cancerous activity	[26]
6	Iron oxide nanoparticle-aptamer bioconjugate	Colon cancer	Epirubicin	Efficiently detect tumors using MRI and reduce cardiotoxicity	[27]
7	Nanostructured lipid carriers	Diabetes	Pioglitazone	Showed significantly extended release in comparison to free form of drug	[28]

Sr. no.	Delivery system	Category	Drug	Outcome	Reference
8	Transdermal patch	Diabetes	Glibenclamide	Better control of hyperglycemia with prolonged plasma half-life	[29]
9	Transniosomes	Parkinson's disease	Thymoquinone	Enhance brain penetration and neuroprotective activity	[30]
10	Niosomes	Parkinson's disease	Bromocriptine	Displaying manifold enhancement in brain distribution and dose reduction upto 10 times	[31]
11	Nanostructured lipid carriers (NLC)	Epilepsy	Diazepam	Achieved nose-to-brain delivery with reduced cytotoxicity	[32]

Table 1.
Examples of smart delivery system.

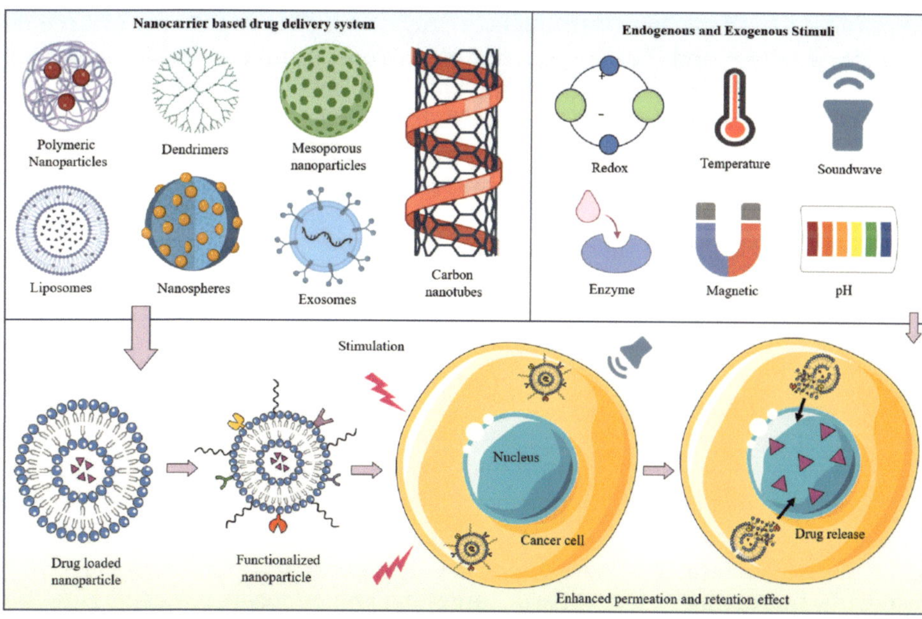

Figure 1.
Different types of stimuli and nanoparticles for the disease management.

3. Future trends and innovations

3.1 Artificial intelligence (AI) and machine learning in drug delivery optimization

Artificial intelligence (AI) and machine learning (ML) have enormous potential in drug discovery, accelerating progress across multiple research disciplines. These tools help to identify new therapeutic targets, better understand disease-target

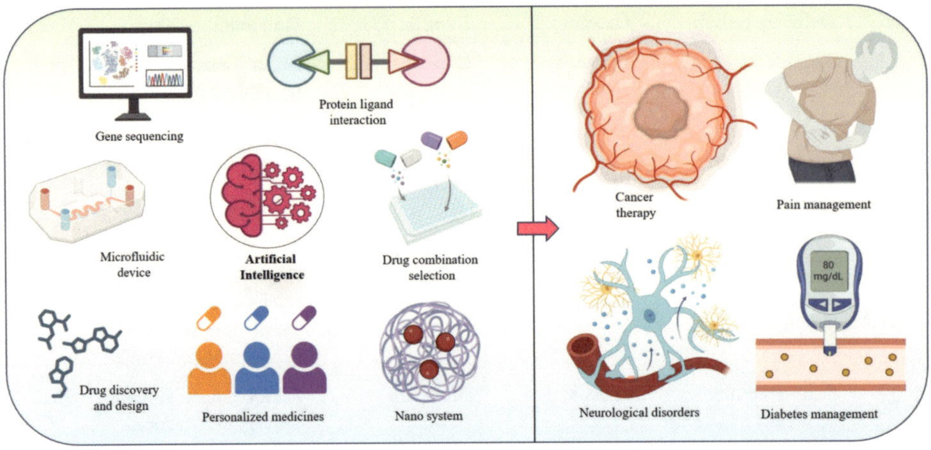

Figure 2.
Future of medicine for the management of diseases like cancer, pain relief, diabetes, and neurological disorders.

relationships, select drug candidates, and predict protein structure (**Figure 2**). Furthermore, AI and machine learning help drug development, a deeper understanding of disease causes, and the identification of prognostic and predictive biomarkers. Moreover, AI and ML are vital in analyzing biometric data *via* wearable devices, precise medicine, and the optimization of clinical trial data. This is especially useful in the global epidemic era when effective data collecting and monitoring at the site are critical to enhancing experimental results [33].

3.2 Gene and mRNA-based therapies

Gene expression regulates protein which is the primary requirement of cellular function. Many diseases are caused by genetic flaws, making gene therapy a viable way of correcting mutations rather than treating symptoms. However, transferring genetic material to specific cells remains difficult because of its degradation and off-target consequences. To improve stability, extend circulation, and enhance targeted distribution, researchers designed specialized DNA delivery and release systems, specifically stimulus-responsive versions. RNA-based medicines, such as siRNA and mRNA, have the potential to treat a variety of conditions when combined with other treatments. Nanocarriers that respond to stimuli improve RNA transport by increasing stability, tissue targeting, and endosomal escape. However, biological variability, undesired off-target effects, complex formulations, and the requirement for specialized activating devices in externally triggered systems all present obstacles [34–36].

3.3 Micro and nanorobots

Micro- and nanorobotic devices are currently being investigated as novel techniques for medicinal delivery in biomedical fields. These devices often pass through and function within a living organism, powered by chemical or bio-hybrid sources [37]. PLA (polylactic acid) and TPU (thermoplastic polyurethane) are biocompatible polymers that are utilized to develop nanorobots and microrobots in medication delivery. These microrobots can navigate complex biological settings by performing controlled motions such as swimming, crawling, or morphing to reach their destinations [38]. They increase drug efficacy by allowing for accurate, immediate release in response to stimuli such as temperature, pH, and magnetic fields. Furthermore, multifunctional designs combine medication administration with sensing or imaging capabilities, which enhances diagnostics and therapy [39].

3.4 Personalized medicine and patient-specific formulation

Personalized medicine is a possible future of healthcare, and smart drug delivery systems (SDDS) will play an important role in its development. Personalized medicine improves treatment efficacy while reducing side effects by modifying drug formulations and optimizing administration based on patient-specific genetic profiles, biomarkers, and factors related to lifestyle. SDDS will eventually combine diagnostic and targeted therapy into a single treatment method. This unique theranostic technique has the potential to offer extremely specific, effective, and accurate treatments for cancer and other persistent diseases, opening the door to personalized chemotherapy with better patient outcomes. Despite their various designs, all smart drug delivery systems goal is to improve patient care [40, 41].

4. Conclusion

The smart delivery system includes stimuli-sensitive delivery systems, controlled drug delivery systems, nanoparticles, and targeted drug delivery systems that are capable of enhancing the therapeutic efficacy of the existing therapeutic moieties. Each of the delivery systems has a defined mechanism to improve the therapeutic efficacy including the targeted release due to internal and external stimuli that increase the drug concentration at the site of action; targeted distribution due to the unique size, ligand-receptor interaction, and abnormal anatomical condition, increase the drug concentration at the site of action; prolong the release of the drug from the delivery system that sustaining minimum therapeutic concentration in the plasma results in the effective management of diseases condition for an extended period of time with reduced toxicity. Overall, the smart drug delivery system effectively manages disease and disorders like cancer, neurological disorders, pain management, infectious diseases, and other chronic disease with their unique mechanism.

Conflict of interest

The authors declare no conflict of interest.

Author details

Rahul Shukla[1*] and Shubhini A. Saraf[2]

1 Department of Pharmaceutics, National Institute of Pharmaceutical Education and Research (NIPER)-Raebareli, Lucknow, Uttar Pradesh, India

2 National Institute of Pharmaceutical Education and Research (NIPER)-Raebareli, Lucknow, UP, India

*Address all correspondence to: rahulshuklapharm@gmail.com; rahul.shukla@niperraebareli.edu.in

References

[1] Fasinu P, Pillay V, Ndesendo VMK, du Toit LC, Choonara YE. Diverse approaches for the enhancement of oral drug bioavailability. Biopharmaceutics & Drug Disposition. 2011;**32**(4):185-209

[2] Tian B, Liu Y, Liu J. Smart stimuli-responsive drug delivery systems based on cyclodextrin: A review. Carbohydrate Polymers. 2021;**251**:116871

[3] Kumar S, Shukla R. Advancements in microneedle technology: Current status and next-generation innovations. Journal of Microencapsulation. 2024;**41**(8):782-803

[4] Jia R, Teng L, Gao L, Su T, Fu L, Qiu Z, et al. Advances in multiple stimuli-responsive drug-delivery systems for cancer therapy. International Journal of Nanomedicine. 2021;**16**:1525-1551

[5] Manzari MT, Shamay Y, Kiguchi H, Rosen N, Scaltriti M, Heller DA. Targeted drug delivery strategies for precision medicines. Nature Reviews Materials. 2021;**6**(4):351-370

[6] Del Amo L, Cano A, Ettcheto M, Souto EB, Espina M, Camins A, et al. Surface functionalization of PLGA nanoparticles to increase transport across the BBB for Alzheimer's disease. Applied Sciences. 2021;**11**(9):4305

[7] Zhang Y, Yang H, Wei D, Zhang X, Wang J, Wu X, et al. Mitochondria-targeted nanoparticles in treatment of neurodegenerative diseases. Exploration. 2021;**1**(3)

[8] Fadnis A, Mhaske A, Shukla R. Neuroprotective potential of Baicalin nanocrystals: Optimisation, comprehensive in vitro SH-SY5Y cell studies and in vivo pharmacokinetics. BioNanoScience. 2025;**15**(2):228

[9] Shukla R, Singh A, Handa M, Flora SJS, Kesharwani P. Nanotechnological approaches for targeting amyloid-β aggregation with potential for neurodegenerative disease therapy and diagnosis. Drug Discovery Today. 2021;**26**(8):1972-1979

[10] Shukla R, Gupta J, Shukla P, Dwivedi P, Tripathi P, Bhattacharya SM, et al. Chitosan coated alginate micro particles for the oral delivery of antifilarial drugs and combinations for intervention in *Brugia malayi* induced lymphatic filariasis. RSC Advances. 2015;**5**(85):69047-69056

[11] Liu P, Chen G, Zhang J. A review of liposomes as a drug delivery system: Current status of approved products, regulatory environments, and future perspectives. Molecules. 2022;**27**(4):1372

[12] Karatas O, Keyikoglu R, Atalay Gengec N, Vatanpour V, Khataee A. A review on dendrimers in preparation and modification of membranes: Progress, applications, and challenges. Materials Today Chemistry. 2022;**23**:100683

[13] de Castro KC, Costa JM, Campos MGN. Drug-loaded polymeric nanoparticles: A review. International Journal of Polymeric Materials and Polymeric Biomaterials. 2022;**71**(1):1-13

[14] Kuperkar K, Patel D, Atanase LI, Bahadur P. Amphiphilic block copolymers: Their structures, and self-assembly to polymeric micelles and polymersomes as drug delivery vehicles. Polymers (Basel). 2022;**14**(21):4702

[15] Anwar M, Muhammad F, Akhtar B. Biodegradable nanoparticles as drug

delivery devices. Journal of Drug Delivery Science and Technology. 2021;**64**:102638

[16] Raza A, Rasheed T, Nabeel F, Hayat U, Bilal M, Iqbal HMN. Endogenous and exogenous stimuli-responsive drug delivery systems for programmed site-specific release. Molecules. 2019;**24**(6):1117

[17] Yu Y, Cheng Y, Tong J, Zhang L, Wei Y, Tian M. Recent advances in thermo-sensitive hydrogels for drug delivery. Journal of Materials Chemistry B. 2021;**9**(13):2979-2992

[18] Ding H, Tan P, Fu S, Tian X, Zhang H, Ma X, et al. Preparation and application of pH-responsive drug delivery systems. Journal of Controlled Release. 2022;**348**:206-238

[19] Zhou Q, Si Z, Wang K, Li K, Hong W, Zhang Y, et al. Enzyme-triggered smart antimicrobial drug release systems against bacterial infections. Journal of Controlled Release. 2022;**352**:507-526

[20] Cheng R, Meng F, Deng C, Klok HA, Zhong Z. Dual and multi-stimuli responsive polymeric nanoparticles for programmed site-specific drug delivery. Biomaterials. 2013;**34**(14):3647-3657

[21] Adepu S, Ramakrishna S. Controlled drug delivery systems: Current status and future directions. Molecules. 2021;**26**(19):5905

[22] Mennini N, Mura P, Nativi C, Richichi B, Di Cesare ML, Ghelardini C. Injectable liposomal formulations of opiorphin as a new therapeutic strategy in pain management. Future Science OA. 2015;**1**(3)

[23] Khanna K, Sharma N, Rawat S, Khan N, Karwasra R, Hasan N, et al. Intranasal solid lipid nanoparticles for management of pain: A full factorial design approach, characterization & gamma scintigraphy. Chemistry and Physics of Lipids. 2021;**236**:105060

[24] Albalawi AE, Alanazi AD, Alyousif MS, Sepahvand A, Ebrahimi K, Niazi M, et al. The high potency of green synthesized copper nanoparticles to prevent the *Toxoplasma gondii* infection in mice. Acta Parasitologica. 2021;**66**(4):1472-1479

[25] Chiappetta DA, Hocht C, Opezzo JA, Sosnik A. Intranasal administration of antiretroviral-loaded micelles for anatomical targeting to the brain in HIV. Nanomedicine. 2013;**8**(2):223-237

[26] Zhou M, Zhao Q, Wu Y, Feng S, Wang D, Zhang Y, et al. Mesoporous carbon nanoparticles as multi-functional carriers for cancer therapy compared with mesoporous silica nanoparticles. AAPS PharmSciTech. 2020;**21**(2):42

[27] Jalalian SH, Taghdisi SM, Shahidi Hamedani N, Kalat SAM, Lavaee P, ZandKarimi M, et al. Epirubicin loaded super paramagnetic iron oxide nanoparticle-aptamer bioconjugate for combined colon cancer therapy and imaging in vivo. European Journal of Pharmaceutical Sciences. 2013;**50**(2):191-197

[28] Ilyas U, Asif M, Wang M, Altaf R, Zafar H, Faran Ashraf Baig MM, et al. Nanostructured lipid carrier-based delivery of pioglitazone for treatment of type 2 diabetes. Frontiers in Pharmacology. 2022;**13**

[29] Mishra MK, Ray D, Barik BB. Microcapsules and transdermal patch: A comparative approach for improved delivery of antidiabetic drug. AAPS PharmSciTech. 2009;**10**(3):928-934

[30] Alkefai NH. Optimization and evaluation of thymoquinone-loaded

transniosome in situ gel for intranasal treatment of Parkinson's disease. Journal of Drug Delivery Science and Technology. 2025;**104**:106565

[31] Sita VG, Jadhav D, Vavia P. Niosomes for nose-to-brain delivery of bromocriptine: Formulation development, efficacy evaluation and toxicity profiling. Journal of Drug Delivery Science and Technology. 2020;**58**:101791

[32] Costa CP, Cunha S, Moreira JN, Silva R, Gil-Martins E, Silva V, et al. Quality by design (QbD) optimization of diazepam-loaded nanostructured lipid carriers (NLC) for nose-to-brain delivery: Toxicological effect of surface charge on human neuronal cells. International Journal of Pharmaceutics. 2021;**607**:120933

[33] Davenport T, Kalakota R. The potential for artificial intelligence in healthcare. Future healthcare Journal. 2019;**6**(2):94-98

[34] Zhou H, Chen DS, Hu CJ, Hong X, Shi J, Xiao Y. Stimuli-responsive nanotechnology for RNA delivery. Advanced Science. 2023;**10**(36)

[35] Xiao Y, Chen J, Zhou H, Zeng X, Ruan Z, Pu Z, et al. Combining p53 mRNA nanotherapy with immune checkpoint blockade reprograms the immune microenvironment for effective cancer therapy. Nature Communications. 2022;**13**(1):758

[36] Zeng H, Zhang Y, Liu N, Wei Q, Yang F, Li J. Stimulus-responsive nanodelivery and release systems for cancer gene therapy: Efficacy improvement strategies. International Journal of Nanomedicine. 2024;**19**:7099-7121

[37] Agrahari V, Agrahari V, Chou ML, Chew CH, Noll J, Burnouf T. Intelligent micro−/nanorobots as drug and cell carrier devices for biomedical therapeutic advancement: Promising development opportunities and translational challenges. Biomaterials. 2020;**260**:120163

[38] Suhail M, Khan A, Rahim MA, Naeem A, Fahad M, Badshah SF, et al. Micro and nanorobot-based drug delivery: An overview. Journal of Drug Targeting. 2022;**30**(4):349-358

[39] Willemen NGA, Morsink MAJ, Veerman D, da Silva CF, Cardoso JC, Souto EB, et al. From oral formulations to drug-eluting implants: Using 3D and 4D printing to develop drug delivery systems and personalized medicine. Bio-Design and Manufacturing. 2022;**5**(1):85-106

[40] Rana A, Adhikary M, Singh PK, Das BC, Bhatnagar S. "Smart" drug delivery: A window to future of translational medicine. Frontiers in Chemistry. 2023;**10**

[41] Boppana SH, Kutikuppala LVS, Sharma S, Madhavrao C, Rangari G, Misra AK, et al. Current approaches in smart nano-inspired drug delivery: A narrative review. Health Science Reports. 2024;7(4)

Chapter 2

Recent Advancement of Nanocrystal Dosage Forms

Jiayi Chen, Zhifeng Zhao, Bhuvanesh Yathavan, Abdur Mirajkar, Dongwei Guo and Jingjun Huang

Abstract

Drug nanocrystal (NC) is a formulation approach, which has been extensively exploited to enhance drug delivery for application in both dissolution rate improvement and sustained release of poorly water-soluble drugs by size reduction and stabilization of the drug particles. Due to the unique physicochemical and pharmacokinetic properties NCs entail, the versatility to be incorporated into various dosage forms for different disease treatments, and the ease of scalability from laboratory development and optimization setting to commercial production by well-developed manufacturing technologies, NCs have attracted tremendous industrial interest, which is reflected by the increasing financial and research and development effort over the last decade. This chapter intends to overview NCs as a viable drug development approach with the introduction on the important aspects of formulation principles and analytical characterizations. The conventional and novel manufacturing methods are highlighted with an emphasis on scalability of widely used wet milling and high-pressure homogenization technologies. The recent application trends of NCs utilized in the pre-clinical studies and clinical trials are discussed further. In addition, the currently marketed products and the future prospective of NCs are elaborated.

Keywords: nanocrystal, nanosuspension, nanoparticles, solubility, bioavailability

1. Introduction

One of the major challenges for the drug development in pharmaceutical industry is the poor solubility of a vast majority of active pharmaceutical ingredients (APIs). Based on the definition of Biopharmaceutical Classification System (BCS), approximately 40% of the currently marketed drugs [1] and as high as 90% of those in the development pipeline [2] are classified as aqueous poorly soluble drugs. The poor solubility generally leads to limited dissolution rate, erratic absorption, and poor bioavailability, which substantially impede the development of new drug products. Many formulation technologies have been exploited to address the solubility issue, which can be classified into two major approaches: (1) to improve the surface area to volume ratio, either by raw drug particles' size reduction or by promoting the porosity, and (2) to modify physicochemical and structural properties by salt formation, cocrystal, solid dispersion, complexation, cyclodextrin inclusion, etc. [3–6], or by a carrier system, such as liposome, nanoemulsion, polymeric or lipid-based nanoparticles, etc [7–10]. However, the second approach usually involves large screening efforts and more complicated preparation methods.

Nanocrystals (NCs) are referred to as carrier-free solid particles of drug substances with a crystalline character in the submicron range, which utilizes the higher surface to volume ratio principle to enhance the dissolution rate and bioavailability. The size reduction is usually achieved by direct crystallization (bottom-up approach) or milling of bulk material (top-down method) [11, 12]. During the manufacturing processes, the microcrystals can also be transformed to amorphous form. As such, in a broad sense, NCs may not be strictly limited to nanoparticles in crystalline form, but sometimes designated as "nanocrystals in the amorphous state". In many cases, NCs are presented as a colloidal dispersion in a media (mostly aqueous) with the help of a stabilizer to prevent/minimize the agglomerations, and therefore they are often regarded as "nanosuspensions" [11, 13, 14]. In this chapter, if not specified, the terms NCs and nanosuspensions are interchangeable.

Besides the common advantages nanosized formulations usually provide, such as increased exposure [15], altered pharmacokinetics (PK) and biodistribution [16], NCs offer unique properties as compared to other feasible formulation approaches, the most eminent being the high drug loading and versatility in terms of administration. Theoretically, NCs can achieve as high as 100% drug loading [17], which tremendously improves efficient drug delivery to target tissue or cellular site at desirable therapeutic concentration. The extremely high drug loading capacity also opens up the possibility of the development of a long-acting drug product [18], which helps to improve patient compliance. In addition, NCs can be delivered by various administration routes, including oral, parenteral, pulmonary, ocular, and topical, which broaden its potential applications.

This chapter overviews NCs as a viable formulation approach outlining the formulation principle and dosage form characterization, the manufacturing methods with recent technology advancement with an emphasis on the scalability, and the recent trends in pre-clinical studies, clinical trials, and marketed products to showcase the broad applications of NCs.

2. Formulation considerations

2.1 Physical stability

Due to the nature of NC, which is composed of an insoluble dispersed phase uniformly distributed throughout a continuous phase, it is classified as a lyophobic colloidal system, which is thermodynamically unstable and tends to aggregate. When larger particles are broken down to smaller ones, work is required to separate the pieces against the forces of attraction between them (ΔW). Hence, the resultant system's Gibbs free energy (ΔG) increases proportionally to the total newly exposed surface area (A), as presented in Eq. (1), wherein γ is the interfacial tension.

$$\Delta G = \Delta W = 2\gamma A \quad (1)$$

The instability of nanosuspensions is commonly manifested as: (1) sedimentation due to an external force, such as gravitation, centrifugation, and electricity; (2) flocculation where the aggregates (flocs) are built up because of the close proximity of the particles and the increasing weak attractive forces, but yet re-dispersible upon shaking to retain the individual particle size or size distribution; (3) caking where the thin liquid film of continuous phase is eliminated from adjacent particles, causing the irreversible formation of larger particles/aggregates; (4) Ostwald ripening, which is a phenomenon associated with polydispersed system of the tendency to one size and ultimately the formation of one large particle, because of the chemical potential and solubility differences between larger and smaller particles.

Successful NC drug product generally depends on the scientist's appreciation for the importance of surface properties of the system. Although NCs are thermodynamically unstable, the interface between the dispersed and continuous phases can be properly treated with stabilizers to generate a repulsive force strong enough to render a kinetically stable system free from aggregation for a sufficient shelf-life. Such interface treatment can be achieved by electrostatic and polymeric methods. Electrostatic stabilization results from charge–charge repulsion, which can be generated by the adsorption of ions from the electrolyte solution, by ionization of the ionizable group, or by selective ion dissolution from particle surface [19, 20]. Polymeric stabilization is achieved by steric stabilization upon adsorption of lyophilic macromolecules at the surface of a lyophobic colloid [21]. In this case, the stabilizing macromolecule needs to be at least a few kilodaltons (kDa) to extend from the surface of the particles over a distance comparable to, or greater than, the distance over which van der Waals attraction is effective. As a result, the colloidal particles will then repel one another because of the volume restriction and osmotic pressure effects. In addition, at low polymer concentrations, and hence low particle surface coverage, lyophilic colloids tend to have multiple points of contact on the lyophobic particle surface and lie along the surface rather than extend from it. This could cause particles to aggregate rather than to repel as the macromolecules adversely adsorb onto multiple particles and thereby bridging flocculation may occur [22].

Nanosuspension stabilizing agents are usually classified into four types: inorganic electrolytes, surfactants, macromolecules, and solid particles [23]. Inorganic electrolytes such as potassium thiocyanate impart a charge at the interface, resulting in electrostatic repulsion between the particles. Surfactants are amphiphilic molecules that reduce the interfacial tension, decrease the contact angle between the particles and the continuous phase, and impart steric stabilization (or charge stabilization in the case of ionic surfactants). Macromolecules, such as synthetic polymers and proteins, function similarly as compared to surfactants, helping to reduce the interfacial tension, and also to form mechanical interfacial barriers. Copolymers with hydrophilic and lipophilic moieties are best with respect to anchoring onto the NC particles. On the other hand, the continuous phase should provide a good solvent environment for the polymer to optimize the stabilization effects.

2.2 Excipients' choice

Besides the stabilizer, other excipients are usually used in NC formulation, including buffering agents, tonicity adjusting agents, antimicrobial preservatives, cryoprotectants, etc. A list of commonly used excipients in an NC drug product is presented in **Table 1**.

Category	Excipient	Common concentration	Example drug product
Stabilizing agent			
Surfactant	Polyoxyethylene sorbitan monooleate (Polysorbate 80)	0.02–2% w/v	Fosaprepitant, Kenalog®, Rapamune®, Ryanodex®
	Polyoxyethylene sorbitan monolaurate (Polysorbate 20)	0.05–1.6% w/v	Invega Sustenna®, Invega Trinza®, Invega Hafyera®, Aristada Initio, Cabenuva, Apretude
	Polyoxyethylene-polyoxypropylene copolymers (Pluronics): Poloxamers 188, 338, and 407	0.1–1% w/v	Rapamune®, Griseofulvin Cabenuva
	Polyoxyl 35 castor oil (Kolliphor EL)	0.4–5% w/v	
	PEG-40 Hydrogenated Castor Oil (Kolliphor RH40)	0.2–2% w/v	
	Polyethylene glycol 15-hydroxystearate (Kolliphor HS 15)	0.25–4% w/v	
	Docusate sodium (SD)	0.25–5% w/v	Megace® ES, Tricor®
	Sodium lauryl sulfate (SLS)	0.02–2% w/v	Emend® (aprepitant), Gris-PEG®, Tricor®, Avinza®, Celebrex®, Griseofulvin
	D-α-tocopheryl polyethylene glycol succinate (TPGS)	0.8–1.5% w/v	
Polymer	Polyvinyl alcohol (PVA)	0.05–1.4% w/v	Tricor®, Rapamune®
	Povidone (PVP)	0.08–1.8% w/v	Tricor®, Rapamune®, Avinza®, Ryanodex®, Celebrex®
	Hypromellose (HPMC)	0.12–1.5% w/v	Megace® ES, Tricor®
	Hydroxyethyl cellulose (HEC)	0.05–0.69% w/v	
	Hydroxypropyl cellulose (HPC)	0.1–0.2% w/v	Emend® (aprepitant)
	Carboxymethylcellulose sodium (CMC-Na)	0.1–0.7% w/v	Kenalog®, Gris-PEG®, Ilevro®
	Polyethylene glycol (PEG) 3350, 4000, and 8000	0.5–3.0% w/v	Cabenuva, Apretude, Invega Sustenna®, Invega Trinza®, Invega Hafyera®, Rapamune®, Focalin XR®
	Microcrystalline cellulose	170–800 mg	Gris-PEG®, Tricor®, Rapamune®, Zanaflex®
Buffering agent	Acetate, Citrate, Tartrate, Phosphate		Megace® ES, Cabenuva Aristada Initio
Tonicity agent	Sodium chloride Glucose Mannitol Dextrose	0.9% w/v 5% w/v 5% w/v 5% w/v	Aristada Initio, Ilevro®, Nevanac® Cabenuva Apretude, Ryanodex®, Nevanac®

Category	Excipient	Common concentration	Example drug product
Preservative	Phenol	0.01–0.75% w/v	Kenalog®
	Metacresol	0.1–0.3% w/v	Gris-PEG®, Griseofulvin
	Benzyl alcohol	0.1–1.0% w/v	Ilevro®, Nevanac®
	Parabens (methyl, propyl, butyl)	0.02–2.0% w/v	Ilevro®
	Benzalkonium chloride	0.01–2.0% w/v	Megace® ES
	Chlorobutanol	0.3–1.1% w/v	
	Thimerosal	0.01–1.0% w/v	
	Phenylmercuric salts (acetate, borate,	0.05–2.0% w/v	
	nitrate)	0.08–5.0% w/v	
	Sodium benzoate		
Cryoprotectant and Bulking Agent	Sucrose	1.0–10% w/v	Tricor®, Rapamune®,
	Mannitol	2.5–7.5% w/v	Griseofulvin
	Trehalose	4–11 mg	Ryanodex®, Somavert®
	Glycine	0.5–200 mg	Somavert®
	Lactose	25–750 mg	Tricor®, Rapamune®,
	Povidone	20–200 mg	Celebrex®
	Sorbitol	1–10% w/v	Colesevelam
	Maltodextrin	3.2–292 mg	hydrochloride
Flavoring agent	Acacia, ginger, anise oil, glucose, benzaldehyde, glycerin, tolu balsam, honey, vanilla, vanilla tincture, lemon oil, clove oil, orange oil, rose oil, fennel oil, coriander oil	0.0001–0.1% w/w	
Coloring agents	Titanium dioxide (white), indigo carmine (blue), tetrazine (yellow), caramel (brown).	0.0005–0.001% w/w	

Table 1.
Commonly used excipients in NC formulation.

2.3 Biopharmaceutical considerations

For nanosuspension absorption from depot sites if by parenteral route, or from intestine if by oral administration, the bioavailability is usually dissolution limited. The rate of dissolution of the drug is governed by the well-known Noyes-Whitney equation:

$$dm/dt = DSh^{-1}(\mathrm{C_s} - \mathrm{C}) \tag{2}$$

where dm/dt is the rate of dissolution, D is the diffusion coefficient of drug in the physiological fluid, S is the surface area of drug exposed to the medium, h represents the thickness of the dissolution layer, C_s is the equilibrium solubility of drug in the physiological fluid, and C is the concentration of drug in that fluid at a given time. Presented by the equation, the dissolution rate can be significantly increased when drug particles are micronized or nanosized. Increased viscosity of the vehicle, for example using oil, could retard drug release because the diffusion coefficient would be expected to decrease in a more viscous medium.

In addition, solubility and bioavailability may also be influenced by the physical state of a drug. When multiple polymorphs exist for NCs, the choice of a crystal form may involve a trade-off between stability and solubility. The choice of a less stable polymorph would be expected to result in higher solubility of the drug, and better bioavailability, but this approach risks conversion of the less stable form to the more stable (less soluble) form during storage.

Furthermore, the bioavailability of NCs can also be impacted by the route of administration (oral, intramuscular, subcutaneous, topical, etc.), the blood flow and/or lymphatic drainage of the administration site, gender, etc. To date, the biofate of NCs remains not fully understood, hence the nanotoxicity has been a major concern. Numerous studies have revealed that there is a relationship between the NCs' route of administration and the downstream cascade of events in order for the specific transporters to carry the NCs to their active sites [11, 24]. In addition, the shape of NCs also plays an important role in dictating the biofate. Generally, the rod-like morphology appeared to penetrate through cells more efficiently as compared to spherically shaped [25, 26]. Alternatively, NCs may undergo transportation via the paracellular pathway, especially when the formulation includes a surfactant such as sodium deoxycholate that is able to open the tight junctions and may facilitate the NCs' penetration, although no tentative evidence is present [27].

3. Manufacturing of NC formulations

3.1 Top-down (Nanonization)

3.1.1 Wet milling

Wet milling, also called media milling, is one of the most commonly used methods to manufacture NC formulations. It decreases the particle size of the active pharmaceutical ingredient (API), which is dispersed in a liquid, via the milling of beads. There are normally four different forces involved in a wet milling process, namely shearing (tearing), impact (crushing), pressure (compression), and attrition (particles tearing and crushing each other) [28]. Different materials of beads, such as glass, steel, zirconium oxide, and polymer resins, have been used as the grinding media. The selection of bead type and bead size depends on the desired product specifications [29]. Wet milling not only reduces the size but also alters the size distribution of the drug particles. Compared to the bulk API, milled drug particles present significantly higher specific surface area. Based on the Noyes-Whitney equation, it will increase the dissolution rate of the milled drug particles [30, 31]. In addition to the size reduction, wet milling also modifies the shape and surface roughness of particles, which is beneficial to the development of inhalable dry powder formulations [32].

Wet milling has many advantages over other nanocrystal formulation fabrication methods, including ease of scale-up, little-to-no yield loss, good versatility, and no involvement of an organic solvent [33]. The major concern of wet milling is the generation of residues from the grinding media that may result in contamination of the final product. However, this issue could be minimized by utilizing highly crosslinked polystyrene resin milling beads [13, 33].

The milling process usually generates lots of heat, affecting further size reduction and crystal formation [34]. In addition, the milled NCs possess a large specific surface area, resulting in increased free energy and decreased thermodynamic stability. Thus, APIs are typically milled together with certain polymers and/or surfactants to prevent agglomeration and to enhance their physical stability, as described in the previous sections [35].

The scalability of a manufacturing process is essential and critical to the success of the development of NC formulations. Wet milling, in this regard, offers full scale-up options from laboratory benchtop instrument for small research and optimization purposes, to commercial production scale equipment (**Table 2**). Hagerdorn et al. investigated the scalability of these milling equipment and they found that DeltaVita 15–300, DeltaVita 600, and DeltaVita 2000–60,000 could generate fully comparable nanoparticles among different batch sizes [35].

3.1.2 High-pressure homogenization

High-pressure homogenization (HPH) applies high pressure when the liquid suspension is passed through a nozzle at high velocity, and the sudden drop of pressure combined with the collision force against the seat valve and impact ring brings about mechanical disruption of the particles [36]. The high-pressure homogenizer could be either a microfluidizer or a piston-gap homogenizer. Microfluidizer employs a Z-type reaction chamber or a Y-type reaction chamber. The Z-type reaction chamber allows the liquid suspension to flow into a Z-shaped channel, generating particle collision and shear forces. While the Y-type reaction chamber separates the drug suspension into two streams, which then collide frontally. The particle size of NCs gets reduced by collision under high pressure and velocity. The piston-gap homogenizers reduce the particle size by shear and collision forces produced during repeat homogenization cycles when the formulation passes through a thin gap [37]. The HPH process is robust and could be easily adapted for aseptic production of parenteral drug formulations. However, metal contamination due to the long duration of homogenization and high-energy production are the main disadvantages associated with HPH [38]. The particle size is unlikely to be reduced to 100 nm by the top-down method. Hence, other methods have been developed to address this issue [39].

Similar to wet milling, high-pressure homogenization is a robust manufacturing method offering equipment for the full range of scales. For example, Microfluidizer® technology-based high-pressure homogenizers not only provide excellent batch-to-batch reproducibility, but also the capability to duplicate results from lab scale to production scale (**Table 3**), thanks to the alignment of microchannels in parallel within the interaction chambers, which ensures that the entire product stream experiences identical shear, regardless of the volume.

Equipment	**DeltaVita 1**	**DeltaVita 15–300**	**DeltaVita 600**	**DeltaVita 2000–60,000**
Batch Size	1–100 mL	35–2000 mL	1–6 L	4–4000 L
Grinding Chamber Volume (mL)	2, 15, 50	15, 50, 150, 300	600	1600, 4000, 10,000, 25,000, 62,000
Grinding Media Diameter (mm)	0.05–2.5	0.05–0.8	0.05–2	0.1–2.0
Drive Power (kW)	2.2	2.2	3	5.5, 15, 18/22, 37/45, 75/90
Speed Range (min^{-1})	—	1000–4200	1000–4500	350–2500
Scale-up	Similar results on all sizes of the DeltaVita series			

Table 2.
Netzsch DeltaVita® grinding technology-based equipment.

Equipment	Benchtop scale			Pilot scale		Production scale
	LV1	LM10	M110P	M110EH	M815	M700 series
Batch Size	1–10 mL	30–300 mL	> 50 mL	120 mL–100 L	1.5–300 L	> 12 L
Operation Pressure (psi)	Up to 30,000	Up to 23,000	Up to 30,000	Up to 30,000	Up to 30,000	Up to 30,000
Flow Rate	—	—	< 120 mL/min	295–450 mL/min	1–1.2 L/min	5–15 L/min
Scale-up	Produce fully comparable results at different scales					

Table 3.
Microfluidizer® technology-based high-pressure homogenizers.

3.2 Bottom-up (Nucleation)

3.2.1 Antisolvent precipitation

The antisolvent precipitation method is a commonly used bottom-up method to generate NCs. In this method, NCs are prepared by mixing a drug solution and an antisolvent to generate high supersaturation, followed by drug precipitation [40, 41]. Typically, stabilizers are used, and they are dissolved in water or antisolvent. The API is dissolved in an organic solvent or solvents. Stabilizers are selected on the basis of their hydrophobic-lipophilic balance (HLB) [42]. Numerous factors, such as the ratio of solvent to antisolvent, stirring speed, stirring time, and stabilizers, could affect the final formulations [43]. This method contains only nucleation and growth steps, so it is simple and cost-effective [44]. However, unstable crystal particles could also be recrystallized in this process, leading to potential aggregation and precipitation of nanocrystals. The other potential issue is solvent residues due to the use of organic solvents in the preparation process. In addition, it is unsuitable for drugs that are neither soluble in aqueous nor insoluble in solvents.

Precipitation assisted by acid-base method is a similar bottom-up method. This method usually involves a weak acid solution dissolving the API as the acid phase, and a weak base solution containing stabilizers as the base phase. The acid phase is slowly added to the base phase to produce carbon dioxide, and then the drug nanocrystals are precipitated by vapor effervescence [45]. This method is applicable only to insoluble drugs with a solubility related to pH and is stable under acid or base. One advantage of this method is that it avoids the usage of organic solvents, which is much more environment-friendly.

3.2.2 Supercritical fluid technology

The supercritical fluid technology utilizes a supercritical fluid (e.g., supercritical carbon dioxide) to dissolve the drug and precipitate NCs with the rapid vaporization of the supercritical fluid as the fluid is atomized under reduced pressure through a nozzle with a tiny aperture [46]. Due to the low polarity of the supercritical fluid, the hydrophobic drug could be easily dissolved and form a solution [47]. Supercritical fluid technology includes rapid expansion of supercritical solution and supercritical antisolvent based on the function of supercritical fluid in the crystallization process. Several parameters contribute to the final particle size of the NCs, including the state of the supercritical fluid in the process, the concentration of the drug, and the morphology of the nozzle. This method does not need organic solvents. However, it consumes large amount of supercritical fluid(s), and it is only suitable for drugs that can be dissolved in supercritical fluids.

4. Recent NCs' technology advancement

4.1 Non-traditional methods

In addition to the well-established and commercially used nanocrystal synthesis methods, there are several innovative and combination technologies by which nanocrystals are prepared in various research laboratories. Herein, we have discussed some of those innovative methods.

Laser ablation is a top-down manufacturing technique commonly used to produce metallic and organic nanoparticles. It involves size reduction by irradiating solids or particles in suspension for nano- or femtoseconds using a laser. A major advantage of laser ablation is the production of stable, contamination-free nanoparticles compared to other commonly utilized technologies [48, 49]. This technique has been successfully applied in synthesizing NCs and holds great potential. Singh et al. [49] used laser ablation to prepare nanocrystals containing three drugs from a pre-formed drug cast on a glass slide. NCs were produced by focusing a femtosecond laser on the cast in liquid. The resulting NCs were stable, free of organic residue, exhibited minimal cytotoxicity, and demonstrated enhanced *in vitro* blood-brain barrier crossing. Similarly, Kenth et al. [48] used femtosecond laser ablation to prepare NCs of poorly soluble paclitaxel. This study explored both ablation and fragmentation aspects of laser technology, as well as the impact of laser power, duration, and focus location on nanocrystal size, drug content, and degradation. Optimal laser power yielded nanocrystals with narrow polydispersity and low degradation. These findings suggest that laser ablation can be used to produce NCs with small drug amounts, providing a valuable tool for preclinical research on new drug entities [48].

Microwave hydrothermal synthesis is a bottom-up manufacturing technique used to produce inorganic NCs for various applications. Recently, this technology has been employed to prepare stable nanocrystals for radiation therapies in cancer treatment. Yi et al. [50] used the microwave hydrothermal technique to prepare hafnium oxide nanocrystals. In their method, hafnium chloride was first heated to 80°C for 1 hour, followed by the addition of sodium hydroxide at room temperature, which was stirred for 30 minutes. The resulting solution was then sealed and placed in a microwave hydrothermal system, where it was heated at a rate of 10°C per minute to 160°C for 1 hour. Afterward, the solution was centrifuged and washed with deionized water, and the precipitate was further modified with polyethylene glycol (PEG) to enhance circulation time and biocompatibility. The synthesized hafnium oxide nano-assembly demonstrated stability in various physiological solutions, making it suitable for parenteral applications. Additionally, the nano-assembly exhibited excellent *in vitro* and *in vivo* antitumor activity in a mouse model [50].

Modified microfluidics has been developed to overcome the limitation of conventional microfluidics method as the conventional T-shaped and Y-shaped microfluidic chips used in this process have limitations in mixing efficiency and require a high percentage of aqueous media for rapid mixing [51]. To address this, Zheng et al. [51]

utilized a split-and-recombine (SAR) chip to improve mixing efficiency and prepare curcumin NCs. In their method, curcumin was dissolved in acetone, while the appropriate stabilizer was dissolved in the aqueous phase. The two solutions were passed through SAR chips to produce a curcumin nanosuspension, which was then centrifuged and washed with deionized water. The resulting curcumin NCs (~60 nm) demonstrated better *in vitro* dissolution and improved oral bioavailability in rats compared to curcumin solution. Given its scalability, microfluidics with SAR chips holds significant potential for the commercial development of drug NCs.

Ultrasonication, either through an ultrasonic bath or through a probe sonicator, is an effective method for reducing particle size and controlling nucleation and crystallization. Ultrasound waves generate cavitation, which enhances heat and mass transfer, resulting in better mixing, creating supersaturation levels, and more controlled nucleation [52]. The factors that influence NC particle size include ultrasound power, sonication time, solution volume, and the probe's diameter and position [53].

Sonication is typically combined with precipitation techniques to achieve the desired NCs. For example, Rahim et al. [54] prepared aceclofenac NCs using a precipitation and sonication method. Aceclofenac was dissolved in ethanol and precipitated into an antisolvent, followed by ultrasonication for varying durations (5, 10, 15, and 20 minutes) and ultrasound power levels (50, 100, 150, 200, 250, and 300 W). The optimal conditions—200 W for 15 minutes—produced stable nanocrystals with the lowest particle size and polydispersity index (PDI). Increasing both the power and sonication time led to an increase in particle size. The batch size was successfully scaled up from 5 mL to 400 mL, addressing one of the common limitations of this technology [54]. Similarly, Xia et al. [55] demonstrated that increasing ultrasonic power and time reduced nanocrystal particle size. However, raising the power beyond 400 W and extending the time beyond 15 minutes did not result in further particle size reduction. Ige et al. [56] successfully utilized probe sonication to prepare stable fenofibrate NCs. Fenofibrate was added to an aqueous solution containing poloxamer 188, and the suspension was stirred at 1000 rpm for 5 minutes to create a homogeneous mixture. The suspension was then subjected to probe sonication at 20–23 kHz for 10 minutes, resulting in stable nanocrystals with a particle size of 420 ± 50 nm and a PDI of 0.458 ± 0.05. Stability studies conducted at 5°C and room temperature over 90 and 180 days showed that the NCs remained stable at both temperatures for 90 days. However, a significant increase in particle size was observed in samples stored at room temperature beyond 90 days, highlighting the need for refrigerated storage.

4.2 Combination technology

Due to the diverse properties of different drugs, there are always limitations of top-down method or bottom-up method. The combination technology selectively unites the top-down technology and the bottom-up technology in a particular sequence, [52, 57] so it overcomes the disadvantages of a single preparation method, and it increases the particle size reduction efficiency. This technology combines a pre-treatment step and a particle size reduction step. It eliminates the drawbacks of instrument clogging and improves the stability of NCs, and it is suitable for a wider range of insoluble drugs. The disadvantages of this technology include high cost and process complexity, thereby using it only when necessary [52]. So far, combinative technology could be divided into the NanoEdge® technology and the SmartCrystal® technology [58, 59].

DOI: http://dx.doi.org/10.5772/intechopen.1007776

4.3 NCs surface modification

Recently, PEGylation of nanocrystals has been used to enhance circulation half-life, improve efficacy, and evade the mononuclear phagocytic system. Zhang et al. [60] reported that PEGylation of paclitaxel nanocrystals not only improved the stability of the nanocrystals during storage and under physiological conditions but also demonstrated superior antitumor activity in breast cancer xenografted mice and lung tumor metastasis models compared to non-PEGylated paclitaxel nanocrystals. These findings highlight the potential significance of PEGylation in future NC research.

NCs are currently used primarily for intravenous administration, with a focus on passive targeting based on their size. However, passive targeting in cancer treatment has limited effectiveness due to the reduced and irregular enhanced permeation and retention (EPR) effect observed in human tumors. The improved efficacy and reduced toxicity seen with active targeting in other nanoparticle technologies, such as liposomes, micelles, and lipid nanoparticles, has driven a recent trend toward surface modification for active targeting in NCs. Active targeting is achieved by attaching a targeting moiety to the nanoparticle surface [59, 61].

For example, Wang et al. demonstrated that hyaluronic acid-coated camptothecin NCs exhibited enhanced anticancer activity in cluster of differentiation 44 (CD44)-overexpressing cell lines and lower toxicity to normal cells compared to free camptothecin and uncoated camptothecin NCs [62]. Gad et al. synthesized docetaxel NCs using pluronic F127 as a stabilizer and albumin as a functional surface modifier. The albumin-coated docetaxel NCs showed improved delivery to multidrug-resistant cell lines compared to free docetaxel [63]. Similarly, Park et al. reported that paclitaxel NCs coated with albumin had an increased plasma half-life, improved tumor deposition, and enhanced anticancer activity compared to Abraxane in a melanoma mouse model [64].

Other surface molecules used for NC targeting include dextran [65], folic acid [66, 67], tocopherol polyethylene glycol 1000 succinate [68], peptides [69], cell membranes [70, 71], and Herceptin [72]. These findings demonstrate the significant potential of surface modification for the targeted delivery of NCs in cancer treatment.

5. NCs characterizations

5.1 Particle size distribution

Particle size distribution (PSD) is a major attribute for NC formulations, therefore particle size measurement is presented to be a critical characterization. The most widely used techniques are elaborated as follows.

Sieve analysis is the traditional method to determine the particle size by stacking several sieves with increasing aperture size. When the material is passed through the stack of sieves, the weight of the material retained by each sieve is recorded as a fraction of the whole mass, and the PSD or gradation is assessed. *Static Image Analysis* (SIA) is predominantly used for measuring narrow size distributions with a focus on the characterization of very fine particles. This method provides high-resolution particle images, which allow for size and shape description with utmost accuracy and are mainly used in research and development applications [73]. *Dynamic Image Analysis* (DIA) describes the particle shape that includes sphericity, symmetry, convexity, and aspect ratio. This method is ideally suited for routine measurements of bulk goods, powders, granules, and suspensions. It is characterized by high sample throughput, reliability, and excellent reproducibility [73]. *Static Laser Light Scattering* (SLS) analysis, also called laser diffraction, is a fast technique providing good flexibility. It could be used to determine whether the native state of a particle is simple or complex and measure the masses of aggregates or other non-native species [74]. *Dynamic Light Scattering* (DLS) is the most versatile and useful set of techniques for measuring the *in situ* size, size distributions, and the shapes of nanoparticles in liquids, which can obtain accurate and statistical particle size distributions (**Table 4**) [75, 76].

5.2 Structural and morphological characterization

The structural characterizations of NCs are critical as they provide important information on the physiochemical properties and stability. X-ray diffraction (XRD) is used to determine the structural parameters and crystal structure of crystalline or amorphous substances [77]. Differential scanning calorimetry (DSC) is a valuable tool to evaluate the thermal behavior of the NCs, such as glass transition temperature, melting point, and associate enthalpy. It could also be used to characterize the interactions between the drug crystals and the excipients [78]. This method is especially useful for the drug product obtained from high-strength top-down processing methods. Fourier transform infrared spectroscopy (FT-IR) method is used to measure the chemical property of the drug crystals and its interaction with different excipients at the molecular level. The change in vibrational frequency of the molecules can exhibit the interaction between different compounds [79]. Thermogravimetric measurements and differential thermal analysis (DTA) are widely applied for NCs thermal analysis. Thermogravimetric analysis is a technique to study the thermal stability, heat flow, and structural deformation of NCs in the inert environment, whereas DTA is used to determine the phase changes and related thermal processes [80].

To characterize the morphological appearance of the drug NCs, scanning electron microscopy (SEM), transmission electron microscopy (TEM), and atomic force microscopy (AFM) are widely applied. SEM and TEM both provide high resolution, being as low as 1 and 0.2 nm, respectively. TEM is usually applied for wet samples and SEM analysis is crucial to monitor the particle shape and size after the process of the water removal. AFM, as a new generation of scanning probe microscopy, is employed to investigate the morphology and surface properties of nanoparticles including height, friction, and magnetism using the scanning probe. A three-dimensional (3D) sample surface image can be obtained by collecting feedback signals from the force

Particle size analysis methods	Size range
Sieve Analysis Dry sieving Wet sieving Air jet sieving	40–125 mm 20–20 mm 10–0.2 mm
Static Image Analysis (SIA)	0.5–1.5 mm
Dynamic Image Analysis (DIA)	1–30 mm
Static Light Scattering (SLS) or Laser Diffraction (LD)	10–4 mm
Dynamic Light Scattering (DLS)	1–10 μm

Table 4.
Suitable size range for different particle size analysis methods.

applied by the probe. More importantly, the shape and structure of NCs is accessible by AFM but not by other methods. A study has revealed that non-spherical shapes significantly outperform their spherical counterparts regarding escaping from phagocytosis and firm binding to the target cells or tissues [81].

5.3 *In vitro* dissolution

In vitro dissolution is employed for drug product quality control and is considered to be a critical tool to predict the *in vivo* performance. It is crucial to select the appropriate dissolution methodology, dissolution conditions, and acceptance criteria not only to assure the product quality but also to evaluate the *in vivo* performance of the drug products.

US Pharmacopeia (USP) methods including paddle or basket apparatus are employed for both orally administered and injectable NC drug products. The dissolution conditions and acceptable criteria can be product specific with different buffers/surfactants to facilitate the NC dissolution. Most of the methods are utilized for quality control purposes, and it is challenging to predict the product's *in vivo* performance. It is difficult to mimic the physiological conditions, which result in the lack of correlation between the *in vitro* dissolution results and *in vivo* bioavailability performance. It is essential to develop an *in vitro-in vivo* correlation (IVIVC), which could be used to surrogate the bioequivalence studies in humans.

Another challenge comes from the separation of undissolved particles from the dissolution medium, which makes it difficult to determine the dissolved drug concentration. In current USP dissolution tests, the different pore size syringe filters are applied to remove the undissolved particles, and it is determined that larger filter sizes could potentially transport smaller sized nanoparticles through the filter membrane, which leads to the dissolution profiles with an apparent supersaturation and large standard deviation. To resolve this problem, the flow cell method is considered to be the most robust dissolution method for NCs and widely employed to evaluate the NC quality attribute and the release of drug *in vitro*. With a constant flow pump, the medium contacts the sample at the lower end of the flow cell at desired temperature and suitable flow rate, the release medium is then filtered through the upper end of the flow cell for dissolved drug measurement [82].

In most cases, the dissolution rate depends on the size and surface area of the NCs. Other parameters including dissolution rate and saturation solubility are also informative to predict the *in vivo* performance of the NCs. To better evaluate the function, metabolism, efficacy, and bioavailability of the drug product, it is still crucial to administer the NC formulations to animals for *in vivo* pharmacokinetic and pharmacodynamic investigations and evaluation.

6. Dosage forms and applications of NCs

6.1 Dosage forms of NCs

NCs present versatility as a formulation approach as they can be formulated into numerous dosage forms, such as tablet and capsules, nanosuspension, dry powder for reconstitution or direct inhalation, etc., and can suit the needs for various routes of administration including oral, parenteral (intravenous, subcutaneous, and intramuscular), pulmonary, ocular, dermal, etc.

Oral administration among all feasible routes is the most compliant and safest route. NCs help to enhance the drug saturation solubility and dissolution rate for absorption. For example, Sirolimus NC formulation developed by Wyeth, the first FDA approved oral NCs, showed 21% higher oral bioavailability than sirolimus solution [83]. Taking another instance, EMEND (Aprepitant oral capsule or suspension) not only enhances oral bioavailability, but also eliminates the food effect, thereby causing no erroneous absorption [84].

Parenteral routes, although require injection thus not as compliable as the oral route, offer irreplaceable advantages regardless. The intravenous (i.v.) route provides 100% bioavailability, hence making it a favorable route for challenging APIs, especially those belonging to class IV drugs of the Biopharmaceutical Classification System (BCS). Research efforts have been made to develop intravenous NC formulations for curcumin [85], ascularine [86], itraconazole [87], and melarsoprol [88]. Subcutaneous (s.c.) and intramuscular (i.m.) routes can be utilized as the depot site for long-acting NCs formulations [89], offering extended drug release, enhanced patient compliance, and cost-effective alternatives for treatment of life-threatening diseases like HIV, as compared to long-term implants [90].

Furthermore, pulmonary [91], ocular [92, 93], and dermal [94] routes have all been studied for local and/or systemic drug delivery by NC formulations.

6.2 Application trends in preclinical and clinical studies

Nanocrystal technology has been widely applied in the development of formulations for poorly soluble drugs, demonstrating its utility across a range of diseases in both preclinical and clinical studies. The application of nanocrystals for various diseases and routes of administration is outlined in **Table 5**. In preclinical trials, parenteral nanocrystals have been explored for treating diseases, such as cancer [64], inflammatory conditions [97], pain management [95], and HIV [99]. Nanocrystals are particularly valuable for improving the solubility of poorly soluble drugs and developing sustained-release formulations, which are advantageous for treating chronic conditions. These sustained-release systems provide a consistent drug dose over an extended period, helping to control the release rate and reduce adverse effects from high drug concentrations.

Several strategies have been employed to overcome challenges related to drug product stability, release kinetics, and *in vivo* behavior. For example, camptothecin nanocrystals, when incorporated into hydrogels and delivered via intra-articular injection for rheumatoid arthritis, showed improved drug residence time and efficacy compared to camptothecin nanocrystals alone [97]. Additionally, Park et al. reported that albumin-coated paclitaxel nanocrystals exhibited an extended plasma half-life, improved tumor deposition, and enhanced anticancer activity compared to Abraxane in a melanoma mouse model [64]. Another promising approach was demonstrated by Liang et al., who incorporated nanocrystals into liposomes. By functionalizing the liposomes with folic acid, they combined the benefits of both technologies, resulting in improved pharmacokinetics, enhanced tumor targeting, and a higher tumor inhibition rate [96].

A search for the term "nanocrystals" on ClinicalTrials.gov identified 24 clinical studies in the past ten years with different routes of administration (**Table 6**). Among those, two were registered for the parenteral route of nanocrystal administration. One study evaluated the safety and efficacy of a 30 mg meloxicam nanocrystal formulation administered through intravenous infusion for the treatment of moderate to

DOI: http://dx.doi.org/10.5772/intechopen.1007776

Drug	Indication	Animal model	Route of adminis-tration	Dose	Stabilizing agent	Reference
Meloxicam	Pain management	Male Sprague–Dawley rats	I.V.	5 mg/kg	Sodium deoxycholate	[95]
CHMFL-ABL-053	Cancer	Male Sprague–Dawley rats	I.V.	1 mg/kg	Pluronic F127; PEG 2000; folic acid	[96]
Camptothecin	Rheumatoid arthritis	Collagen-induced arthritis rat model	I.V.	1.3 mg CPT/ml	α-Tocopherol	[97]
Cabotegravir	HIV	Healthy male Sprague–Dawley rats	I.M.	40 mg/kg	Polysorbate 20 and polyethylene glycol 3350	[98]
Atazanavir	HIV	BALB/cJ mice chronic infection model	I.M.	50 mg/kg	Folic acid and poloxamer 407	[99]
Nintedanib	Non-small cell lung cancer	Healthy Sprague–Dawley rats	Oral	62 μg/mL	Sodium carboxyl methyl cellulose	[100]
Acetazolamide	Glaucoma, ocular hypertension	Steroid glaucoma Albino rabbit model	Ophthalmic	0.2%w/v (100 μl)	Poly-γ-glutamic acid and hyaluronic acid	[101]
Mometasone furoate	Allergic rhinitis and rhinosinusitis	Male mice	Nasal	0.05 w/v % (2 μL)	Two-hydroxypropyl-β-cyclodextrin and methylcellulose	[102]
Fusidic acid	Wound infection	Rat excision wound infection model	Topical	2% (w/w)	PVA 4–88	[103]
Glibenclamide	Hyperglycemia	Male Albino rats diabetic model	Pulmonary	34 μg	Polyvinylpyrrolidone 30	[104]

Table 5.
Selected nanocrystals preclinical trials in the last five years.

NCT Number	Indication	Drug	Sponsor	Route of administration	Trial phase	Start year
NCT06408727	Amyotrophic Lateral Sclerosis	CNM-Au8	Clene Nanomedicine	Oral	NA	
NCT06379165	Pain	Meloxicam Nanocrystal Injection	CSPC ZhongQi Pharmaceutical Technology Co., Ltd.	I.V.	Phase 3	2023
NCT05541107	Cryptococcal Meningitis	MAT2203	Matinas BioPharma	Oral	Phase 3	2023
NCT04299386	Dental Implant Failure Nos	NeoPhylaxis	Université de Montréal		NA	2023
NCT05437731	Orbital Deformity	Coated titanium mesh	Hams Hamed Abdelrahman	Orbital reconstruction	NA	2022
NCT05299658	Amyotrophic Lateral Sclerosis	CNM-Au8	Clene Nanomedicine	Oral	Phase 2	2021
NCT05281484	Amyotrophic Lateral Sclerosis	CNM-Au8	Clene Nanomedicine	Oral		2022
NCT04675242	Blepharitis	NCX 4251	Nicox Ophthalmics, Inc.	Ophthalmic	Phase 2	2020
NCT04626921	Relapsing Multiple Sclerosis	CNM-Au8	Clene Nanomedicine	Oral	Phase 2, 3	2020
NCT04156152	Hypersensitivity Dentin	Nanocrystals of Hydroxyapatite toothpaste	Universidad del Desarrollo		NA	2020
NCT03843710	Amyotrophic Lateral Sclerosis	Gold Nanocrystals	Clene Nanomedicine	Oral	Phase 2	2020
NCT04203056	Schizophrenia	Aripiprazole Lauroxil	University of California, Los Angeles	I.M.	Phase 4	2019
NCT04098406	Amyotrophic Lateral Sclerosis	CNM-Au8	Clene Nanomedicine	Oral	Phase 2	2019
NCT04091256	Dentinal Hypersensitivity	Zinc-carbonate Hydroxyapatite Nanocrystals	Qassim University		NA	2019
NCT04081714	Multiple Sclerosis	CNM-Au8	Clene Nanomedicine	Oral		
NCT03993171	Multiple Sclerosis	Gold nanocrystals	Clene Nanomedicine	Oral	Phase 2	2019

DOI: http://dx.doi.org/10.5772/intechopen.1007776

NCT Number	Indication	Drug	Sponsor	Route of administration	Trial phase	Start year
NCT03926026	Blepharitis	Fluticasone Propionate Nanocrystal	Nicox Ophthalmics, Inc.	Ophthalmic	Phase 2	2019
NCT03815916	Parkinson's Disease	Gold Nanocrystals	Clene Nanomedicine	Oral	Phase 2	2019
NCT03980847	Bone Resorption	Nanocrystalline hydroxyapatite	Islamic Azad University, Tehran		Phase 2	2018
NCT03536559	Relapsing Multiple Sclerosis	CNM-Au8	Clene Nanomedicine	Oral	Phase 2	2018
NCT04376060	Horizontal Ridge Deficiency	Gen-Os®; The soft lamina (OsteoBiol®)	Saint-Joseph University	Bone regeneration	NA	2017
NCT02629419	Candidiasis, Chronic Mucocutaneous	Amphotericin B	Matinas BioPharma Nanotechnologies, Inc.	Oral	Phase 2	2016
NCT02755870	Healthy Volunteers - Male and Female	CNM-Au8	Clene Nanomedicine	Oral	Phase 1	2015
NCT02365675	Pemphigus, Pemphigoid	Nanocrystalline silver (Acticoat)	Fundación Nacional para la Enseñanza y la Investigación de la Dermatología A.C.	Topical	NA	2015

**The database at ClinicalTrials.gov was accessed on October 2nd, 2024.*

Table 6.
Nanocrystals in the clinical trial over the last decade.*

Trade Name	Active ingredient	Indication	Administration route	Company	Approval year
Emend	Aprepitant	Antiemetic	Oral	Merck	2003
Apretude	Cabotegravir	Anti-HIV	I.M.	ViiV Healthcare	2021
Celebrex	Celecoxib	Anti-inflammatory	Oral	G.D. Searle	1998
Ryanodex	Dantrolene sodium	Skeletal muscle relaxant	I.V.	Eagle Pharma	2014
Focalin XR	Dexmethylphenidate hydrochloride	Antipsychotic	Oral	Novartis	2008
Tricor	Fenofibrate	Hypercholesterolemia	Oral	Abbott	2004
Triglide	Fenofibrate	Hypercholesterolemia	Oral	Skye Pharma	2005
Gris-PEG	Griseofulvin	Antifungal infection	Oral	Novartis	1998
Megace ES	Megestrol acetate	Anti-anorexic	Oral	Par Pharma	2005
Ritalin LA	Methylphenidate hydrochloride	Antipsychotic	Oral	Novartis	2002
Avinza	Morphine sulfate	Antichronic pain	Oral	Elan Pharma	2000
Cesamet	Nabilone	Antiemetic	Oral	Lilly	2006
Naprelan	Naproxen sodium	Anti-inflammatory	Oral	Elan Pharma	1996
Ilevro	Nepafenac	Anti-inflammatory	Ocular	Alcon Research	2012
Invega Sustenna	Paliperidone palmitate	Antidepressant	I.M.	Johnson & Johnson	2009
Rapamune	Rapamycin/ Sirolimus	Immunosuppressive	Oral	Wyeth	1999
Zanaflex	Tizanidine hydrochloride	Muscle relaxant	Oral	Elan Pharma	2002
Verelan PM	Verapamil	Antihypertensive	Oral	Elan Pharma	1998

Table 7.
List of selected NC-based marketed products.

severe pain (NCT06379165). Another studycompared the efficacy of a long-acting injectable antipsychotic drug in a nanocrystal formulation with an oral antipsychotic drug to prevent relapse following an initial episode of schizophrenia (NCT04203056). The low number of clinical trials underscores the need for further research to address challenges related to parenteral product stability and *in vivo* efficacy. To overcome these challenges during drug development and improve clinical outcomes, nanocrystals can be combined with other technologies, such as liposomes, *in situ* gels, and polymeric surface coatings [105].

6.3 Commercial products

A list of selected NC-based commercial products is presented in **Table** 7. It is clear that the currently successful NC-based products are mainly indicated for anti-infections and antipsychotic. They focus on addressing the poor drug bioavailability of the existing drug or aiming to provide extended release profile for drugs of frequent and chronic use.

7. Conclusion and perspectives

As compared to other nanotechnology-based formulation approaches, such as liposome, polymeric or lipid-based solid nanoparticles, nanoemulsions, NC offers unique advantages, particularly the ease of scale-up, extremely high drug loading (up to 100%), the versatility for different dosage forms, and the capability of being tailored into a long-acting drug product. Since the first new drug application (NDA) of Gris-PEG (griseofulvin ultramicrosize) back in 1973, a rising trend can be seen for the development and use of NCs [13]. The submissions for NCs drug products comprise approximately 30% of all the applications in the recent two decades, implying the explosive blossoming of NCs development. These submissions cover a wide range of treatment indications and route of administration/dosage forms of NCs drug products. Currently, over 20 products are being marketed and many more will enter the market in the foreseeable future.

To fully utilize the potential of NCs, a few aspects have been suggested [17]: (1) To use NCs not only beyond the predominantly studied solubility enhancer, but also as a drug delivery system for other small molecular drugs or macromolecules to be anchored onto the crystals; (2) to understand in depth the underlying mechanism of NCs cellular uptake and *in vivo* fate; (3) to develop hybrid NCs with environment-sensitive dyes for bio-imaging purpose; and (4) to systematically assess NCs pharmacokinetics, biodistribution, targeting effect, biocompatibility, immunogenicity, therapeutic efficacy, and toxicity *in vivo*.

Acknowledgements

The authors acknowledge Dr. Shaukat Ali for his valuable suggestions.

Conflict of interest

The authors declare no conflict of interest.

Author details

Jiayi Chen*, Zhifeng Zhao, Bhuvanesh Yathavan, Abdur Mirajkar, Dongwei Guo and Jingjun Huang
Ascendia Pharmaceuticals, Inc., North Brunswick, New Jersey, United States

*Address all correspondence to: jiayi.chen@ascendiapharma.com

References

[1] Chogale MM, Ghodake VN, Patravale VB. Performance parameters and characterizations of nanocrystals: A brief review. Pharmaceutics. 2016;**8**(3)

[2] Price DJ, Nair A, Kuentz M, Dressman J, Saal C. Calculation of drug-polymer mixing enthalpy as a new screening method of precipitation inhibitors for supersaturating pharmaceutical formulations. European Journal of Pharmaceutical Sciences. 2019;**132**:142-156

[3] Kumar S, Bhargava D, Thakkar A, Arora S. Drug carrier systems for solubility enhancement of BCS class II drugs: A critical review. Critical Reviews in Therapeutic Drug Carrier Systems. 2013;**30**(3):217-256

[4] Kalepu S, Nekkanti V. Insoluble drug delivery strategies: Review of recent advances and business prospects. Acta Pharmaceutica Sinica B. 2015;**5**(5):442-453

[5] Sanghvi R, Evans D, Yalkowsky SH. Stacking complexation by nicotinamide: A useful way of enhancing drug solubility. International Journal of Pharmaceutics. 2007;**336**(1):35-41

[6] Janssens S, Van den Mooter G. Review: Physical chemistry of solid dispersions. The Journal of Pharmacy and Pharmacology. 2009;**61**(12):1571-1586

[7] Couvreur P, Tulkens P, Roland M, Trouet A, Speiser P. Nanocapsules: A new type of lysosomotropic carrier. FEBS Letters. 1977;**84**(2):323-326

[8] Crommelin DJ, Storm G. Liposomes: From the bench to the bed. Journal of Liposome Research. 2003;**13**(1):33-36

[9] Singh Y, Meher JG, Raval K, Khan FA, Chaurasia M, Jain NK, et al. Nanoemulsion: Concepts, development and applications in drug delivery. Journal of Controlled Release. 2017;**252**:28-49

[10] Muller RH, Shegokar R, Keck CM. 20 years of lipid nanoparticles (SLN and NLC): Present state of development and industrial applications. Current Drug Discovery Technologies. 2011;**8**(3):207-227

[11] Muller RH, Gohla S, Keck CM. State of the art of nanocrystals--special features, production, nanotoxicology aspects and intracellular delivery. European Journal of Pharmaceutics and Biopharmaceutics. 2011;**78**(1):1-9

[12] Shegokar R, Muller RH. Nanocrystals: Industrially feasible multifunctional formulation technology for poorly soluble actives. International Journal of Pharmaceutics. 2010;**399**(1-2):129-139

[13] Chen ML, John M, Lee SL, Tyner KM. Development considerations for nanocrystal drug products. The AAPS Journal. 2017;**19**(3):642-651

[14] Moschwitzer JP. Drug nanocrystals in the commercial pharmaceutical development process. International Journal of Pharmaceutics. 2013;**453**(1):142-156

[15] Patel VR, Agrawal YK. Nanosuspension: An approach to enhance solubility of drugs. Journal of Advanced Pharmaceutical Technology & Research. 2011;**2**(2):81-87

[16] Lu Y, Qi J, Dong X, Zhao W, Wu W. The in vivo fate of nanocrystals. Drug Discovery Today. 2017;**22**(4):744-750

[17] Mohammad IS, Hu H, Yin L, He W. Drug nanocrystals: Fabrication methods and promising therapeutic applications. International Journal of Pharmaceutics. 2019;**562**:187-202

[18] Surve DH, Jindal AB. Recent advances in long-acting nanoformulations for delivery of antiretroviral drugs. Journal of Controlled Release. 2020;**324**:379-404

[19] Sun B, Yeo Y. Nanocrystals for the parenteral delivery of poorly water-soluble drugs. Current Opinion in Solid State & Materials Science. 2012;**16**(6):295-301

[20] Du J, Li X, Zhao H, Zhou Y, Wang L, Tian S, et al. Nanosuspensions of poorly water-soluble drugs prepared by bottom-up technologies. International Journal of Pharmaceutics. 2015;**495**(2):738-749

[21] Morozova TI, Lee VE, Panagiotopoulos AZ, Prud'homme RK, Priestley RD, Nikoubashman A. On the stability of polymeric nanoparticles fabricated through rapid solvent mixing. Langmuir. 2019;**35**(3):709-717

[22] Burgess DJ. Physical stability of dispersed systems. In: Burgess DJ, editor. Injectable Dispersed Systems. Boca Raton, FL: CRC Press; 2019. pp. 1-37

[23] Tadros TF, B. V. Emulsion stability. In: PB, editor. Encyclopedia of Emulsion Technology. 1. New York: Dekker; 1983. pp. 130-278

[24] Rejman J, Oberle V, Zuhorn IS, Hoekstra D. Size-dependent internalization of particles via the pathways of clathrin- and caveolae-mediated endocytosis. The Biochemical Journal. 2004;**377**(Pt 1):159-169

[25] Chaurasiya B, Huang L, Du Y, Tang B, Qiu Z, Zhou L, et al. Size-based anti-tumoral effect of paclitaxel loaded albumin microparticle dry powders for inhalation to treat metastatic lung cancer in a mouse model. International Journal of Pharmaceutics. 2018;**542**(1-2):90-99

[26] Oh N, Park JH. Endocytosis and exocytosis of nanoparticles in mammalian cells. International Journal of Nanomedicine. 2014;**9**(Suppl 1):51-63

[27] Sakai M, Imai T, Ohtake H, Azuma H, Otagiri M. Effects of absorption enhancers on the transport of model compounds in caco-2 cell monolayers: Assessment by confocal laser scanning microscopy. Journal of Pharmaceutical Sciences. 1997;**86**(7):779-785

[28] Merisko-Liversidge E, Liversidge GG, Cooper ER. Nanosizing: A formulation approach for poorly-water-soluble compounds. European Journal of Pharmaceutical Sciences. 2003;**18**(2):113-120

[29] Juhnke M, Martin D, John E. Generation of wear during the production of drug nanosuspensions by wet media milling. European Journal of Pharmaceutics and Biopharmaceutics. 2012;**81**(1):214-222

[30] Li F, Li L, Wang S, Yang Y, Li J, Liu D, et al. Improved dissolution and oral absorption by co-grinding active drug probucol and ternary stabilizers mixtures with planetary beads-milling method. Asian Journal of Pharmaceutical Sciences. 2019;**14**(6):649-657

[31] Hattori Y, Haruna Y, Otsuka M. Dissolution process analysis using model-free Noyes-Whitney integral equation. Colloids and Surfaces. B, Biointerfaces. 2013;**102**:227-231

[32] Chaurasiya B, Zhao YY. Dry powder for pulmonary delivery: A comprehensive review. Pharmaceutics. 2020;**13**(1)

[33] Jacob S, Nair AB, Shah J. Emerging role of nanosuspensions in drug delivery systems. Biomaterials Research. 2020;**24**:3

[34] Ho R, Naderi M, Heng JY, Williams DR, Thielmann F, Bouza P, et al. Effect of milling on particle shape and surface energy heterogeneity of needle-shaped crystals. Pharmaceutical Research. 2012;**29**(10):2806-2816

[35] Hagedorn M, Liebich L, Bogershausen A, Massing U, Hoffmann S, Mende S, et al. Rapid development of API nano-formulations from screening to production combining dual centrifugation and wet agitator bead milling. International Journal of Pharmaceutics. 2019;**565**:187-198

[36] Ferreira A, Figueiredo D, Ferreira F, Ribeiro B, Reis A, da Silva TL, et al. Impact of high-pressure homogenization on the cell integrity of tetradesmus obliquus and seed germination. Molecules. 2022;**27**(7)

[37] Pinar SG, Oktay AN, Karakucuk AE, Celebi N. Formulation strategies of nanosuspensions for various administration routes. Pharmaceutics. 2023;**15**(5)

[38] Krause KP, Kayser O, Mader K, Gust R, Muller RH. Heavy metal contamination of nanosuspensions produced by high-pressure homogenisation. International Journal of Pharmaceutics. 2000;**196**(2):169-172

[39] Salazar J, Ghanem A, Muller RH, Moschwitzer JP. Nanocrystals: Comparison of the size reduction effectiveness of a novel combinative method with conventional top-down approaches. European Journal of Pharmaceutics and Biopharmaceutics. 2012;**81**(1):82-90

[40] Ahmadi Tehrani A, Omranpoor MM, Vatanara A, Seyedabadi M, Ramezani V. Formation of nanosuspensions in bottom-up approach: Theories and optimization. Daru. 2019;**27**(1):451-473

[41] Wu CY, Wang W. Application of antisolvent precipitation method for formulating excipient-free nanoparticles of psychotropic drugs. Pharmaceutics. 2022;**14**(4)

[42] Elmowafy M, Shalaby K, Al-Sanea MM, Hendawy OM, Salama A, Ibrahim MF, et al. Influence of stabilizer on the development of luteolin nanosuspension for cutaneous delivery: An In vitro and In vivo evaluation. Pharmaceutics. 2021;**13**(11)

[43] Awan AM, Farid A, Shah SU, Khan D, Ur Rehman F, Dar MJ, et al. Nanocrytals-mediated oral drug delivery: Enhanced bioavailability of amiodarone. Pharmaceutics. 2022;**14**(6)

[44] Thanh NT, Maclean N, Mahiddine S. Mechanisms of nucleation and growth of nanoparticles in solution. Chemical Reviews. 2014;**114**(15):7610-7630

[45] Han X, Wang M, Ma Z, Xue P, Wang Y. A new approach to produce drug nanosuspensions CO_2-assisted effervescence to produce drug nanosuspensions. Colloids and Surfaces. B, Biointerfaces. 2016;**143**:107-110

[46] Misra SK, Pathak K. Supercritical fluid technology for solubilization of poorly water soluble drugs via micro- and naonosized particle generation. ADMET DMPK. 2020;**8**(4):355-374

[47] Park H, Kim JS, Kim S, Ha ES, Kim MS, Hwang SJ. Pharmaceutical applications of supercritical fluid extraction of emulsions for micro-/nanoparticle formation. Pharmaceutics. 2021;**13**(11)

[48] Kenth S, Sylvestre JP, Fuhrmann K, Meunier M, Leroux JC. Fabrication of paclitaxel nanocrystals by femtosecond laser ablation and fragmentation. Journal of Pharmaceutical Sciences. 2011;**100**(3):1022-1030

[49] Singh A, Kutscher HL, Bulmahn JC, Mahajan SD, He GS, Prasad PN. Laser ablation for pharmaceutical nanoformulations: Multi-drug nanoencapsulation and theranostics for HIV. Nanomedicine. 2020;**25**:102172

[50] Li Y, Qi Y, Zhang H, Xia Z, Xie T, Li W, et al. Gram-scale synthesis of highly biocompatible and intravenous injectable hafnium oxide nanocrystal with enhanced radiotherapy efficacy for cancer theranostic. Biomaterials. 2020;**226**:119538

[51] Zheng X, Zhang J, Zhang L, Huangfu X, Li Y, Chen J. Controlled preparation of curcumin nanocrystals by detachable stainless steel microfluidic chip. International Journal of Pharmaceutics. 2024;**663**:124574

[52] Fontana F, Figueiredo P, Zhang P, Hirvonen JT, Liu D, Santos HA. Production of pure drug nanocrystals and nano co-crystals by confinement methods. Advanced Drug Delivery Reviews. 2018;**131**:3-21

[53] Chan HK, Kwok PC. Production methods for nanodrug particles using the bottom-up approach. Advanced Drug Delivery Reviews. 2011;**63**(6):406-416

[54] Rahim H, Sadiq A, Khan S, Khan MA, Shah SMH, Hussain Z, et al. Aceclofenac nanocrystals with enhanced in vitro, in vivo performance: Formulation optimization, characterization, analgesic and acute toxicity studies. Drug Design, Development and Therapy. 2017;**11**:2443-2452

[55] Xia D, Quan P, Piao H, Piao H, Sun S, Yin Y, et al. Preparation of stable nitrendipine nanosuspensions using the precipitation-ultrasonication method for enhancement of dissolution and oral bioavailability. European Journal of Pharmaceutical Sciences. 2010;**40**(4):325-334

[56] Ige PP, Baria RK, Gattani SG. Fabrication of fenofibrate nanocrystals by probe sonication method for enhancement of dissolution rate and oral bioavailability. Colloids and Surfaces. B, Biointerfaces. 2013;**108**:366-373

[57] Pardhi E, Vasave R, Srivastava V, Yadav R, Mehra NK. Nanocrystal technologies in biomedical science: From the bench to the clinic. Drug Discovery Today. 2024;**29**(3):103913

[58] Soliman KA, Ibrahim HK, Ghorab MM. Effects of different combinations of nanocrystallization technologies on avanafil nanoparticles: In vitro, in vivo and stability evaluation. International Journal of Pharmaceutics. 2017;**517**(1-2):148-156

[59] Ahire E, Thakkar S, Darshanwad M, Misra M. Parenteral nanosuspensions: A brief review from solubility enhancement to more novel and specific applications. Acta Pharmaceutica Sinica B. 2018;**8**(5):733-755

[60] Zhang H, Hu H, Zhang H, Dai W, Wang X, Wang X, et al. Effects of PEGylated paclitaxel nanocrystals on breast cancer and its lung metastasis. Nanoscale. 2015;**7**(24):10790-10800

[61] Lu L, Xu Q, Wang J, Wu S, Luo Z, Lu W. Drug nanocrystals for active tumor-targeted drug delivery. Pharmaceutics. 2022;**14**(4)

[62] Wang J, Muhammad N, Li T, Wang H, Liu Y, Liu B, et al. Hyaluronic acid-coated camptothecin nanocrystals for targeted drug delivery to enhance anticancer efficacy. Molecular Pharmaceutics. 2020;**17**(7):2411-2425

[63] Gad SF, Park J, Park JE, Fetih GN, Tous SS, Lee W, et al. Enhancing docetaxel delivery to multidrug-resistant cancer cells with albumin-coated nanocrystals. Molecular Pharmaceutics. 2018;**15**:871-881

[64] Park J, Park JE, Hedrick VE, Wood KV, Bonham C, Lee W, et al. A comparative In vivo study of albumin-coated paclitaxel nanocrystals and abraxane. Small. 2018;**14**(16):e1703670

[65] Shegokar R, Singh KK. Surface modified nevirapine nanosuspensions for viral reservoir targeting: In vitro and in vivo evaluation. International Journal of Pharmaceutics. 2011;**421**(2):341-352

[66] Talekar M, Ganta S, Amiji M, Jamieson S, Kendall J, Denny WA, et al. Development of PIK-75 nanosuspension formulation with enhanced delivery efficiency and cytotoxicity for targeted anti-cancer therapy. International Journal of Pharmaceutics. 2013;**450**(1-2):278-289

[67] Liu F, Park JY, Zhang Y, Conwell C, Liu Y, Bathula SR, et al. Targeted cancer therapy with novel high drug-loading nanocrystals. Journal of Pharmaceutical Sciences. 2010;**99**(8):3542-3551

[68] Choudhury H, Gorain B, Pandey M, Kumbhar SA, Tekade RK, Iyer AK, et al. Recent advances in TPGS-based nanoparticles of docetaxel for improved chemotherapy. International Journal of Pharmaceutics. 2017;**529**(1-2):506-522

[69] Shubar HM, Dunay IR, Lachenmaier S, Dathe M, Bushrab FN, Mauludin R, et al. The role of apolipoprotein E in uptake of atovaquone into the brain in murine acute and reactivated toxoplasmosis. Journal of Drug Targeting. 2009;**17**(4):257-267

[70] Fan Y, Hao W, Cui Y, Chen M, Chu X, Yang Y, et al. Cancer cell membrane-coated nanosuspensions for enhanced chemotherapeutic treatment of glioma. Molecules. 2021;**26**(16)

[71] Fan Y, Cui Y, Hao W, Chen M, Liu Q, Wang Y, et al. Carrier-free highly drug-loaded biomimetic nanosuspensions encapsulated by cancer cell membrane based on homology and active targeting for the treatment of glioma. Bioactive Materials. 2021;**6**(12):4402-4414

[72] Noh JK, Naeem M, Cao J, Lee EH, Kim MS, Jung Y, et al. Herceptin-functionalized pure paclitaxel nanocrystals for enhanced delivery to HER2-postive breast cancer cells. International Journal of Pharmaceutics. 2016;**513**(1-2):543-553

[73] Fernández-Caballero A, Gómez FJ, López-López J. Road-traffic monitoring by knowledge-driven static and dynamic image analysis. Expert Systems with Applications. 2008;**35**(3):701-719

[74] Kaasalainen M, Aseyev V, von Haartman E, Karaman DS, Makila E, Tenhu H, et al. Size, stability, and porosity of mesoporous nanoparticles characterized with light scattering. Nanoscale Research Letters. 2017;**12**(1):74

[75] Brar SK, Verma M. Measurement of nanoparticles by light-scattering techniques. TrAC Trends in Analytical Chemistry. 2011;**30**(1):4-17

[76] Lim J, Yeap SP, Che HX, Low SC. Characterization of magnetic nanoparticle by dynamic light scattering. Nanoscale Research Letters. 2013;**8**(1):381

[77] Young TJ, Mawson S, Johnston KP, Henriksen IB, Pace GW, Mishra AK. Rapid expansion from supercritical to aqueous solution to produce submicron suspensions of water-insoluble drugs. Biotechnology Progress. 2000;**16**(3):402-407

[78] Danley RL. New heat flux DSC measurement technique. Thermochimica Acta. 2002;**395**(1-2):201-208

[79] Hu L, Kong D, Hu Q, Gao N, Pang S. Evaluation of high-performance curcumin nanocrystals for pulmonary drug delivery

both in vitro and in vivo. Nanoscale Research Letters. 2015;**10**(1):381

[80] Jahangir MA, Imam SS, Muheem A, Chettupalli A, Al-Abbasi FA, Nadeem MS, et al. Nanocrystals: Characterization overview, applications in drug delivery, and their toxicity concerns. Journal of Pharmaceutical Innovation. 2020;**17**:237-248

[81] Daum N, Tscheka C, Neumeyer A, Schneider M. Novel approaches for drug delivery systems in nanomedicine: Effects of particle design and shape. Wiley Interdisciplinary Reviews. Nanomedicine and Nanobiotechnology. 2012;**4**(1):52-65

[82] Yuan-biao X, Peng-fei Y, Ji-xiu D, Jun-nan X, Qin Z, Ming Y. Research progress of in vitro release evaluation methods for nano preparation. Chinese Pharmaceutical Journal. 2016;**51**(11):861-866

[83] Kesisoglou F, Panmai S, Wu Y. Nanosizing--oral formulation development and biopharmaceutical evaluation. Advanced Drug Delivery Reviews. 2007;**59**(7):631-644

[84] Wu Y, Loper A, Landis E, Hettrick L, Novak L, Lynn K, et al. The role of biopharmaceutics in the development of a clinical nanoparticle formulation of MK-0869: A beagle dog model predicts improved bioavailability and diminished food effect on absorption in human. International Journal of Pharmaceutics. 2004;**285**(1-2):135-146

[85] Gao Y, Li Z, Sun M, Guo C, Yu A, Xi Y, et al. Preparation and characterization of intravenously injectable curcumin nanosuspension. Drug Delivery. 2011;**18**(2):131-142

[86] Ganta S, Paxton JW, Baguley BC, Garg S. Formulation and pharmacokinetic evaluation of an asulacrine nanocrystalline suspension for intravenous delivery. International Journal of Pharmaceutics. 2009;**367**(1-2):179-186

[87] Rabinow B, Kipp J, Papadopoulos P, Wong J, Glosson J, Gass J, et al. Itraconazole IV nanosuspension enhances efficacy through altered pharmacokinetics in the rat. International Journal of Pharmaceutics. 2007;**339**(1-2):251-260

[88] Ben Zirar S, Astier A, Muchow M, Gibaud S. Comparison of nanosuspensions and hydroxypropyl-beta-cyclodextrin complex of melarsoprol: Pharmacokinetics and tissue distribution in mice. European Journal of Pharmaceutics and Biopharmaceutics. 2008;**70**(2):649-656

[89] Shi Y, Lu A, Wang X, Belhadj Z, Wang J, Zhang Q. A review of existing strategies for designing long-acting parenteral formulations: Focus on underlying mechanisms, and future perspectives. Acta Pharmaceutica Sinica B. 2021;**11**(8):2396-2415

[90] Kirby T. Long-acting injectable for HIV approved for use in the UK. The Lancet Infectious Diseases. 2022;**22**(1):26

[91] Britland S, Finter W, Chrystyn H, Eagland D, Abdelrahim ME. Droplet aerodynamics, cellular uptake, and efficacy of a nebulizable corticosteroid nanosuspension are superior to a micronized dosage form. Biotechnology Progress. 2012;**28**(5):1152-1159

[92] Ali HS, York P, Ali AM, Blagden N. Hydrocortisone nanosuspensions for ophthalmic delivery: A comparative study between microfluidic nanoprecipitation and wet milling. Journal of Controlled Release. 2011;**149**(2):175-181

[93] Gupta S, Samanta MK, Raichur AM. Dual-drug delivery system based on in situ gel-forming nanosuspension of forskolin to enhance antiglaucoma

efficacy. AAPS PharmSciTech. 2010;**11**(1):322-335

[94] Yu Q, Wu X, Zhu Q, Wu W, Chen Z, Li Y, et al. Enhanced transdermal delivery of meloxicam by nanocrystals: Preparation, in vitro and in vivo evaluation. Asian Journal of Pharmaceutical Sciences. 2018;**13**(6):518-526

[95] Ma L, He Y, Bai L, Li M, Sui X, Liu B, et al. Preclinical studies of a high drug-loaded meloxicam nanocrystals injection for analgesia. Colloids and Surfaces. B, Biointerfaces. 2022;**218**:112777

[96] Liang H, Zou F, Liu Q, Wang B, Fu L, Liang X, et al. Nanocrystal-loaded liposome for targeted delivery of poorly water-soluble antitumor drugs with high drug loading and stability towards efficient cancer therapy. International Journal of Pharmaceutics. 2021;**599**:120418

[97] Gao Y, Vogus D, Zhao Z, He W, Krishnan V, Kim J, et al. Injectable hyaluronic acid hydrogels encapsulating drug nanocrystals for long-term treatment of inflammatory arthritis. Bioengineering & Translational Medicine. 2022;**7**(1):e10245

[98] Jucker BM, Alsaid H, Rambo M, Lenhard SC, Hoang B, Xie F, et al. Multimodal imaging approach to examine biodistribution kinetics of cabotegravir (GSK1265744) long acting parenteral formulation in rat. Journal of Controlled Release. 2017;**268**:102-112

[99] Puligujja P, Balkundi SS, Kendrick LM, Baldridge HM, Hilaire JR, Bade AN, et al. Pharmacodynamics of long-acting folic acid-receptor targeted ritonavir-boosted atazanavir nanoformulations. Biomaterials. 2015;**41**:141-150

[100] Zhu Y, Fu Y, Zhang A, Wang X, Zhao Z, Zhang Y, et al. Rod-shaped nintedanib nanocrystals improved oral bioavailability through multiple intestinal absorption pathways. European Journal of Pharmaceutical Sciences. 2022;**168**:106047

[101] Donia M, Osman R, Awad GAS, Mortada N. Polypeptide and glycosaminoglycan polysaccharide as stabilizing polymers in nanocrystals for a safe ocular hypotensive effect. International Journal of Biological Macromolecules. 2020;**162**:1699-1710

[102] Masuda S, Deguchi S, Ogata F, Yoshitomi J, Otake H, Kanai K, et al. Nasal absorption enhancement of mometasone furoate nanocrystal dispersions. International Journal of Nanomedicine. 2023;**18**:5685-5699

[103] Ahmed IS, Elnahas OS, Assar NH, Gad AM, El Hosary R. Nanocrystals of fusidic acid for dual enhancement of dermal delivery and antibacterial activity: In vitro, ex vivo and In vivo evaluation. Pharmaceutics. 2020;**12**(3)

[104] Alotaibi MR, Fatani AJ, Almnaizel AT, Ahmed MM, Abuohashish HM, Al-Rejaie SS. In vivo assessment of combined effects of glibenclamide and losartan in diabetic rats. Medical Principles and Practice. 2019;**28**(2):178-185

[105] Rossier B, Jordan O, Allemann E, Rodriguez-Nogales C. Nanocrystals and nanosuspensions: An exploration from classic formulations to advanced drug delivery systems. Drug Delivery and Translational Research. 2024;**14**:3438-3451

Chapter 3

Nanoengineered Microneedles: A Versatile Targeted Delivery System for Theragnostic Applications

Mansi Singh and Rahul Shukla

Abstract

Microneedles (MNs) have been used as active drug delivery carriers by precisely delivering drugs to the targeted site along with minimal tissue destruction. Earlier, MNs were used for the delivery of drugs to the transdermal site; now they are used as drug delivery carriers to the solid tumor site, mucosal, ophthalmic, and other organ site-specific drug delivery. MNs are considered a boon for trans-barrier delivery because other drug delivery routes, such as systemic and parenteral, face challenges by limiting the optimum amount of drug reaching the skin or other barrier-containing organs. Hence, MN-mediated drug delivery enhances permeation and improves brain and transdermal delivery of drugs by ciliary nasal clearance and crossing the nasal barrier. The current book chapter mainly focuses on the recent advancements in the area of MN-based drug delivery carriers into various parts of the body, their theragnostic applications, mainly the organs containing barriers, and encounters with delivery challenges has been discussed. Also, the comprehensive overview of MN types, fabrication polymers, mechanisms of drug release, effectiveness, and advantages over conventional delivery systems have been summarized.

Keywords: MNs, nanoformulations, therapeutics, diagnostics, MN types, drug delivery

1. Introduction

Nanoengineered MNs are an innovative approach in the field of theragnostic, which blends therapeutic and diagnostic features on a single platform. These sophisticated MNs include nanotechnology to boost their efficiency, providing a diverse and successful way for targeted medication delivery and application in diagnosis [1]. MNs are tiny threads that range in length from 50 to 950 mm and are meant to penetrate the skin's outermost layer, the corneal layer, without reaching nerve endings. This enables medicine delivery with the least discomfort and minimal suffering. Nanoengineering upgrades this technology by adding nanomaterials (NMs) and precision manufacturing methods, resulting in increased performance and versatility [2]. Arguably the most notable benefit of nanoengineered MNs is their ability to deliver medication with pinpoint accuracy. Traditional medication delivery strategies, such as oral or intravenous ingestion, frequently encounter problems such as variable absorption rates, systemic adverse effects, and compliance from patient issues. MNs, on the other hand, can avoid these issues by dispensing drugs in a limited and regulated manner [3]. MNs can be constructed to transport a variety of therapeutic agents, including small-molecule medicines and biologics like vaccines and monoclonal antibodies [4]. The use of MNs facilitates the development of MNs with superior mechanical properties, drug-encapsulating information, and controlled release profiles. For example, biodegradable polymer MNs can release therapeutic payloads over time, eliminating the requirement for frequent administration [5]. Alongside medication administration, nanoengineered MNs are making great progress in diagnostic applications. These MNs can be equipped with nanosensors or functionalized with specific molecules to detect biomarkers linked to certain diseases. This integration allows for real-time monitoring of physiological parameters and early diagnosis of illnesses, including diabetes, infection, and cancer [6]. MNs fitted with glucose sensors, for example, can provide diabetic patients with continuous glucose monitoring, giving them real-time input on their blood sugar levels and eliminating the need for repeated finger pricking [7]. Similarly, MNs loaded with antibodies can identify specific bacteria or cancer signals in interstitial fluid, which may offer a less intrusive and more accessible way of detection than traditional blood testing [8].

2. The versatility of nanoengineered MNs

i. Multimodal delivery systems - Nanoengineered MNs have been constructed to perform numerous functions concurrently, making them extremely versatile; for example, MNs can be designed to deliver a combination of pharmaceuticals and diagnostic chemicals [9]. This dual capacity is especially valuable in situations when monitoring and therapy must be synchronized. MNs array might administer a drug while collecting samples for diagnostic tests, such as measuring glucose levels in diabetic patients or tracking blood biomarkers for chronic conditions [7].

ii. Tailored drug release -The architecture of nanoengineered MNs permits highly adjustable medication release characteristics. Researchers can construct controlled mechanisms for drug delivery by altering the material and structure of MNs—either slowly over time or in response to specific physiological cues [10]. This adaptability is useful for treating chronic illnesses that require sustained release, such as hormone therapies or anticancer medication. In contrast, MNs can be developed for quick release in emergency conditions, providing customized therapeutic responses [11].

iii. Difficult but hands-off solution - MNs provide a noninvasive complement to typical injection procedures, which reduces patient discomfort and boosts compliance. The precision of MNs ensures that just the outer layer of skin is penetrated, avoiding nerve endings and reducing pain. This noninvasive property qualifies MNs for use in immunization, cosmetic treatment, and continuous health monitoring, all of which prioritize patient comfort [12].

iv. Customized medicine - MNs may be tailored to suit each patient's specific needs, which is a key component of personalized treatment. MNs, for example, can be programmed to give drug doses tailored to each person's genetic or metabolic profile. This technique improves treatment efficacy while avoiding side effects by tailoring the drug delivery mechanism to each patient's specific needs [13].

3. Manufacturing methods for creating MN-based thermosensors

Micro-Electro-Mechanical Systems (MEMS) are the most promising technology for creating perfect MN designs since it allows MNs to be manufactured accurately and uniformly to make precision devices. Originally, MNs were created by etching arrays of micron-sized needles into silicon using standard microfabrication techniques [14]. They were then developed using a range of materials, including metals like titanium and stainless steel as well as ceramic, glass, polydimethylsiloxane (PDMS), dextrin, and polymers [15]. Other techniques utilized in the production of MNs include laser cutting, micro-molding, 3D printing, lithography, photolithography, and cutting [16]. MN types in various therapeutic applications are explained graphically in **Figure 1**.

3.1 3D printing

MNs' commercialization and clinical applications have been delayed because of the high cost and intricate synthesis processes [17]. As a result, not only can MNs be fabricated using the 3D printing technology in a single step (print and fill), but personal customization is also feasible [15]. This method, which creates MNs with a variety of forms and geometries, is based on a computer-aided drug creation model that puts the material selectively layer by layer [18]. A range of 3D printing techniques, including sheet lamination, photopolymerization, material extrusion, powder bed fusion, and binder jetting, is provided to create adaptable MNs for a variety of uses in the medical field [19].

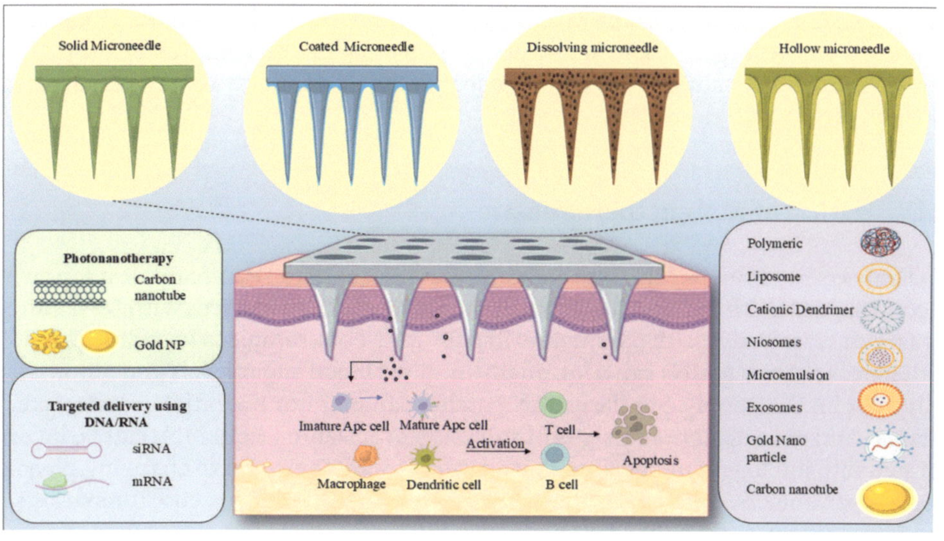

Figure 1.
MN types in various therapeutic applications.

3.2 Photolithography

Photolithographic processes in microelectronic technology require spin-coating a liquid photosensitive polymer, called photographs resist, onto a substrate, which is subsequently heated to a solid state. After that, the photoresist is exposed to UV light through a mask, simulating the structure's design [20]. Typically, a design is made (known for the main pattern) and is utilized to build a pattern of holes by replicating it onto a thin substrate, usually a silicon wafer [21]. It uses a UV-visible light radiation source to transfer a predetermined shape from the photomask to the substrate, which is often coated beforehand with a photosensitive substance, in order to create hollow MNs [22].

3.3 Etching

This technique involves slicing exposed portions of solid material with a strong liquid (acid) or by hand in order to create a pattern [23]. Dry and wet etching are two of the various etching procedures; the use depends on the building material and the kind of MNs to be produced [24]. While gas is used in dry etching, which is more costly and necessitates techniques like vapor phase or plasma etching, the wet etching technique uses a liquid to remove the layers from the MN's surface to create the desired shape [25]. MNs were created in a study by utilizing a dry reactive ion etching method with a chromium masking substance [26].

3.4 Cutting

Using CAD software, solid MNs are laser-cut to the required size and shape for the fabrication of stainless steel sheets. This hard material (silicon) MN production process is rarely widely employed since the product deteriorates due to the equipment's metal blades [27]. MNs are created by electropolishing, which speeds up drug permeation and minimizes the amount of time needed for MN insertion, or by manually bending the MN structure after metal has been cut with an infrared laser [28]. The beam adopts the shape of a needle, cleaning the needle with hot water and bending it at a 90-degree angle before electropolishing it with compressed air to reduce its breadth or sharpen its tips. Consequently, this method—known as 3D laser cutting—uses a laser to cut [19].

4. Utilization of MNs in theragnostic

The incorporation of MNs into wearable devices marks a significant development in continuous health monitoring. Smart patches or wearable devices with MNs can measure a variety of health parameters in real time. For example, a wearable patch with glucose-sensing MNs can continually monitor blood sugar levels and automatically alter insulin supply. Similarly, MN patches can monitor hydration, electrolyte balance, and even detect early signs of infection or inflammation. MNs can be incorporated into intelligent medication delivery devices that respond to changing physiological parameters. MNs embedded with sensors might detect specific biomarkers and release medication only when necessary [29].

This clever strategy guarantees that medication is administered precisely when needed, optimizing therapeutic outcomes and reducing unnecessary drug exposure.

MNs can perform both diagnostic and therapeutic activities in a single device, resulting in a comprehensive theragnostic tool. The device could be built to detect cancer biomarkers while also administering targeted treatment. This integration enables real-time monitoring of disease progression and quick therapeutic action, which improves treatment efficacy and patient outcomes. The use of MNs in remote health monitoring systems contributes to the emerging field of telemedicine. MN-based devices can collect health information and send it to healthcare specialists for remote analysis. This capacity is especially useful for controlling chronic disease or for remote and underserved locations where access to healthcare institutions may be restricted [30]. In an emergency, MNs can provide quick, on-demand remedies. MNs developed for administering emergency drugs, epinephrine for anaphylaxis, or naloxone for opioid overdose, can be delivered swiftly. MNs are perfect for integrating into first-aid kits or emergency response equipment due to their small size and ease of use. Snakebite infestation is a WHO priority neglected disease that causes numerous local and systemic harmful consequences. Recent research has found certain pharmacological targets that, when administered parentally. Based on the information that is at present accessible, it is hypothesized that a formulation of treatments applied internally through convenient, self-administered MNs will either hinder the lymphatic drainage transit and absorption of HMw venom toxins into the bloodstreams or inhibit the mechanistic pathway of LMw toxins. This formulation might thus be more beneficial for pre-hospital management shortly after a snakebite than PBI alone [31].

5. Advanced design and functionality

i. NM integration - The use of NM with MN technology has greatly improved its performance. Material including gold NPs, carbon nanotubes, and silica NPs are used to change the physical and chemical properties of MNs. These materials lead to several significant improvements [32]. NPs can encapsulate medications more effectively than traditional approaches. They enable regulated release profiles, which involve delivering medication at a consistent pace over time or in response to specified stimuli. This is especially useful for treatments that require prolonged release, such as hormone therapy or vaccinations. NM can increase MN's mechanical strength and flexibility, making them less likely to break or bend during insertion. Silicon-based MNs can be coated with tiny layers of NMs to improve endurance while retaining sharpness for efficient penetration. The functionalization of nanoparticles enables tailored medication delivery. Drugs can be precisely delivered to the cells or tissues of interest by attaching specific ligands or antibodies to MNs. This targeting lowers off-target effects while increasing treatment efficacy [33].

ii. MN array - MNs can be assembled in a variety of arrangements, such as arrays or patches, to increase their functionality. Arrays are made up of several MNs placed in a grid pattern, allowing for the delivery of multiple drugs at the same time or complete interstitial fluid sampling [34]. Advanced MN arrays are designed to penetrate various skin levels, enabling both superficial and deeper drug administration [35].

iii. Self-dissolving MNs - They are a novel approach to MN technology. These are constructed of biocompatible materials that disintegrate after being inserted into the skin, releasing the drug payload. This removes the need for needle removal, lowers the danger of infection or discomfort, and makes the procedure more convenient for patients. Researchers created sdMN and found that this approach has great immunization effectiveness in both mice and humans. To understand the process of immune response induction, which is the basis for the efficiency and safety [36].

6. Current advancements in nanoengineered MNs

Nanoengineered MNs represent an evolutionary shift in biomedical technology, providing novel options for therapeutic and diagnostic purposes. These innovative technologies, distinguished by their small size and exquisite engineering, are on the verge of changing healthcare by combining minimal invasiveness with high efficiency [27]. This thorough examination dives into current breakthroughs in nanoengineered MNs, emphasizing their diverse roles in modern medicine and their potential to influence the future of healthcare. Diagnostic-therapeutic potential of MNs is given in **Table 1.**

6.1 Therapeutic approach

i. Vaccine delivery - The development of nanoengineered MNs has transformed vaccine delivery, overcoming various constraints associated with traditional vaccination methods [52]. Traditional vaccine administration, often by intramuscular injections, is often uncomfortable and needs competent staff. MNs represent a promising option that is both less intrusive and maybe more effective. MNs improve vaccine administration by forming microchannels in the skin's outer layer, allowing antigens to interact directly with immune cells in the epidermis and dermis. This interaction may result in a stronger immunological response than typical injection approaches. Studies have shown that MN-based vaccine delivery can dramatically improve vaccine immunogenicity, as seen by better immune responses to influenza and hepatitis B vaccines. One of the most distinguishing qualities of MNs is their ease of use. MN patches can be self-administered, decreasing the requirement for healthcare personnel and increasing vaccine availability. This trait is especially useful in mass immunization efforts and remote places where healthcare services are limited [53]. MN patches have been demonstrated to improve vaccination coverage and compliance due to their ease of usage. Recent advancements include MNs intended for COVID-19 vaccinations, which have demonstrated encouraging effects in preclinical trials. These MNs not only administer the vaccine effectively, but they also stimulate a powerful immune response while minimizing pain and suffering. Current clinical trials are evaluating the effectiveness of MN-based vaccines in real-world conditions.

ii. Drug delivery - The creation of nanoengineered MNs had a significant impact on drug delivery, opening up new opportunities for precise and regulated administration of medicinal substances [54]. MNs can be designed to release medications at a controlled rate, which is critical for therapies that require continuous or scheduled release. For example, MNs constructed of biodegradable polymers

S.No.	MNs	Material/ Therapeutics	Disease	Outcome	Reference
1	5- amino levulinate-dissolving MN patches	Sodium hyaluronate	Cancer	Tips loaded with 5-aminolevulinic MNs demonstrated a higher melanoma inhibitory rate (97%) than parenteral formulation (66%) when compared to injectable formulation. This is because of the unique properties of MNs, which allow the drug to be delivered at the appropriate time and amount by creating microchannels in the skin, increasing the drug's bioavailability.	[37]
2	Hydrogel MN patch	HA	Diabetes	Showed regulated release throughout a 24-hour period, while the oral dosage only produced a 4-hour therapeutic effect.	[38]
3	Dissolvable MN	HA	Rheumatoid arthritis	Transepidermal drug delivery, which enhances biocompatibility and has strong anti-inflammatory efficacy in mice	[39]
4	MN patch	HA	Obesity	More effective than the traditional technique, the delivery of caffeine along with HA in the form of an MN patch enhances the solubility of caffeine in the formulation and inhibits crystal formation.	[40]
5	Hydrogel MN	HA	Rheumatoid arthritis	In 90% of mice, the creation of hydrogel MN for DTA6 administration showed an improvement in aptamer stability for up to 72 hours, protecting the joints and bones from erosion in collagen-induced arthritis.	[41]
6	DissolvingMN		Obesity	A research study created MN of rosiglitazone, a browning agent that, because of the presence of a β-3 adrenoreceptor agonist that releases the medication gradually, changes WAT into BAT for the treatment of obesity.	[42]

S.No.	MNs	Material/ Therapeutics	Disease	Outcome	Reference
7	Solid MNs		Neurological disorder	In one study, topical 4% lidocaine cream displayed its therapeutic effect after 60 minutes, but pretreatment of the skin with solid MNs loaded with lidocaine generated anesthesia in just 30 minutes.	[43]
8	Dissolving MNs		Neurological disorder	Some transdermal local anesthetics (bupivacaine, lidocaine, etc.] blocked sodium channels and resulted in numbness in the skeletal muscles when applied repeatedly. By releasing MNs patches into the affected area, CGRP8–37, an anti-CGRP peptide, was administered without systemic exposure or negative effects.	[44]
9	Stainless steel MN	Pilocarpine	Ophthalmic	According to a study, injecting stainless steel MN laden with pilocarpine intrasclerally increased the absorption rate by 45 times.	[45]
10	Hollow MNs	Sulforhodamine	Ophthalmic	Hollow MNs combined with sulforhodamine; the MN array was created using borosilicate micropipette tubes, which have a 10–35 μL drug administration limit.	[46]
11	Dissolvable MNs	Artemether and lumefantrine	Malaria	The preferred treatments for malaria are lumefantrine (LUM) and artemether (ART), yet they have drawbacks such as hydrophobicity and poor oral absorption. In order to improve bioavailability, dissolvable MNs containing the medication in micro-suspension were created, and MN-LUM was shown to be more effective in controlling transdermal administration than oral therapy.	[47]

S.No.	MNs	Material/ Therapeutics	Disease	Outcome	Reference
12	MNs array	Artemether co-loaded lumefantrine nanoparticles	Malaria	The MNs array was created by the solvent casting process with co-loaded lumefantrine nanoparticles loaded with artemether. The study showed that the array was completely permeated, showing drug release up to 60–70% with a 6-month stability period that extended the release to 24 hours. Therefore, when it came to transepidermal distribution of BCS class II and IV medicines, MNs outperformed oral administration in terms of efficiency and safety.	[48]
13	Swellable MNs	HA	Ophthalmic	Swellable MNs aided by methacrylate HA (MEHA) were created to quickly extract almost 1.4 mg of ISF for the detection of metabolites like hyperglycemia and cholesterol.	[37]
14	Hydrogel MNs	Poly-l-lysine	Malaria	The skin's immunological cells are tracked by multifunctional antibodies (MNs). For example, the skin was treated with Poly-l-lysine MNs, which have an alginate hydrogel surface coated in immunological adjuvants and antigens. Leukocytes penetrate the hydrogel layer, activate the adjuvants present in the MN, and attract T-cells for additional analysis. Another study used hydrophilic hollow MNs (MNs) to rapidly identify protein biomarkers in interstitial fluid, particularly Plasmodium falciparum histidine-rich protein 2, a biomarker for malaria.	[49]

S.No.	MNs	Material/ Therapeutics	Disease	Outcome	Reference
15	MN-based sensors	Iridium oxide layer	Infection	To detect in vivo concentrations of β-lactam antibiotics, MN-based biosensors are coated with a pH-sensitive iridium oxide layer on the electrode surface. These biosensors are stable and sterilizable for up to two weeks at 20°C. The lactamase enzyme mounted on the electrode surface hydrolyzes the lactam ring, causing a change in local pH that the biosensor measures.	[50]
16	Coated MNs	PDMS	Ophthalmic	Showed that traditional MNs placed in people for extended periods of time have a danger of breaking due to stress or motion; as a result, researchers created and assessed porous, PDMS matrix MN with an HA coating. Additionally, they demonstrated the effectiveness of flexible MNs in collecting ISF via compression for ongoing glucose monitoring both in vitro and in vivo (mouse).	[51]
17	MN array	PLGA	Rheumatoid arthritis	To treat RA, a methotrexate-loaded MN array with PLGA microspheres of folic acid was developed to boost methotrexate's bioavailability and allow for dosage reduction.	[38]

Table 1.
Diagnostic-therapeutic potential of MNs.

can gradually release medications over time, reducing the frequency of administration [34]. This method has been used for hormone therapy, such as insulin delivery for diabetes control, in which maintaining consistent medication levels is critical for optimal treatment. The detachable dissolving MNs (DDMNs) have an array of needles that can be removed using the administration of the foundation sheet. Here, researchers were established to tackle the problems of insulin storage stability and delivery efficiency [55]. More theragnostic application of MNs using NIR irradiation to treat tumors is explained in **Figure 2**.

MNs have a huge benefit in that they may deliver drugs to places within the body. Drugs can be delivered to specific cells or tissues, such as cancer cells or inflammatory

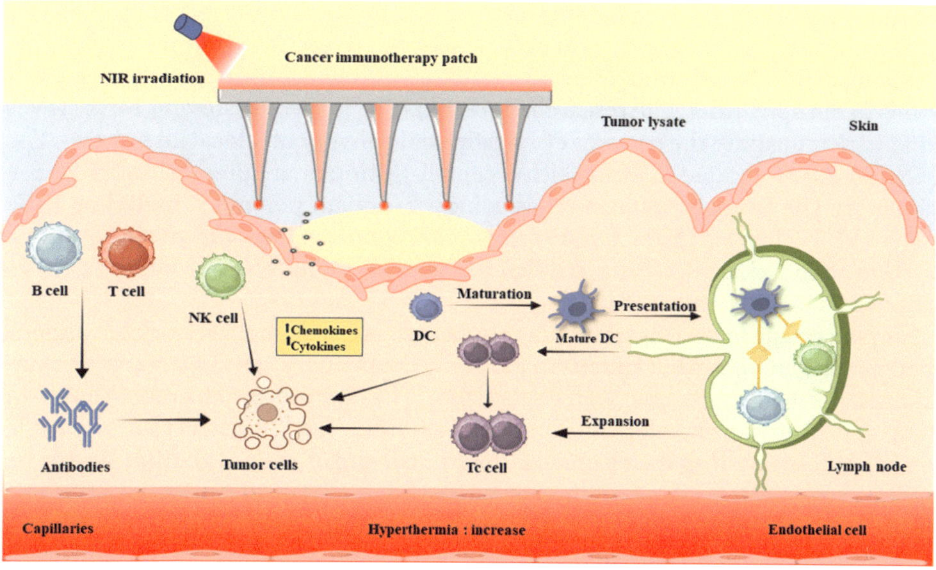

Figure 2.
Theragnostic application of MNs using NIR irradiation to treat tumors.

areas, by loading MNs with targeting ligands or antibodies. This focused strategy reduces systemic exposure and potential negative effects, which improves therapeutic efficacy. For example, MNs coated with antibodies targeting tumor-specific antigens have demonstrated potential in delivering chemotherapeutic drugs directly to cancer cells [56].

MNs have been studied for localized pain relief, providing an alternative to systemic pain medicines. MNs administer analgesics directly to the source of pain, resulting in localized alleviation with minimal systemic effects. This method is especially useful for controlling chronic pain problems like arthritis, when traditional pain management strategies may be ineffective or have substantial adverse effects. Castilla-Casadiego et al. developed and tested a chitosan MN patch for transdermal delivery of meloxicam to treat pain in cattle. Chitosan and chitosan/meloxicam MN patches were assessed for chemical composition, physical homogeneity, skin penetration, and thermal and thermo-mechanical reaction. MN patches were made with varied acetic acid concentrations: 92 (v/v), 52 (v/v), and 15% (v/v). Additionally, drug release was evaluated by modeling varying percentages of skin penetration and the number of MNs on the patch. Scanning electron microscopy confirmed that MNs were equally distributed on the patch surface for each proportion of acetic acid applied. The MN patches successfully penetrated the skin in a cow's cadaver ear. The average depth of penetration assessed following complete dehydration of the penetrated skin was 78 ± 1 μm. Higher acetic acid percentages in chitosan and chitosan/meloxicam MN patches resulted in increased compressive force resistance at higher temperatures [57].

Recent innovations include MN patches that deliver anti-inflammatory medicines or local anesthetics transdermally. These patches provide a noninvasive and effective solution to treat problems such as dermatitis and post-surgical discomfort. The development of MNs for hormone replacement therapy demonstrates their usefulness in treating a variety of chronic illnesses. Ropivacaine hydrochloride (RPL) is a local anesthetic commonly used to alleviate pain during or after surgery. However, this medicine is only accessible in parenteral form and may aid in the infiltration of RPL into the plasma, resulting in certain unwanted side effects. Intradermal delivery of RPL using dissolving MNs could be a promising technique for delivering such medications to the epidermis. The researcher created RPL-loaded dissolving MNs (DMN-RPLs) to demonstrate the concept of intradermal delivery of a local anesthetic. The DMN-RPLs were created utilizing either centrifugation or air-pressurized chamber techniques. The DMN-RPLs were made using a variety of polymers, including PVP, PVA, and SH. Thermal characteristics, chemical bonding, mechanical strength, insertion ability, skin-dissolving studies, and drug content were all evaluated on the manufactured DMN-RPLs [58].

For ocular delivery - The sclera is a matrix embedded with a network of randomly ordered collagen fibers that functions as one of the primary static barriers of the eye and prevents drug molecules from penetrating. The choroid-Bruch's membrane, the sclera, and pigments like melanin all operate as strong static barriers that prevent big molecules from entering the vitreous humor or the site of action. To improve the penetration of medications through tissues, numerous permeation enhancers have been studied. These compounds' primary drawback is that they irritate the tissues of the eyes, and there are still concerns about biocompatibility and ocular safety. Physical elements like iontophoresis or sonication can improve the penetration of medications through the sclera [25]. The principles of cavitation and vibration underlie sonication's operation. The disintegration of polymeric MNs may be aided or accelerated by the vibrations produced during sonication. As a result, it helps medicines penetrate the sclera more quickly. Iontophoresis improves the electrostatic force-driven molecular diffusion in a similar manner. Enhancing and controlling the flow of molecules across the barrier is largely dependent on the electrical charge on the molecules. In the presence of an electric charge, iontophoresis increases the penetration of ionized substances through the sclera. These techniques in conjunction with MNs would improve macromolecule penetration, including oligopeptides, peptides, and proteins [59].

iii. Cosmetic applications - MNs have applications beyond traditional medicine, including dermatological and cosmetic therapies. Their capacity to improve the delivery of skincare products has created new opportunities for boosting skin health and beauty. MNs are utilized to administer anti-aging medicines such as retinoids, peptides, and HA straight to the skin. This method improves the penetration and activity of these compounds, resulting in enhanced skin texture and fewer indications of aging. MN-based delivery devices have been shown in studies to greatly boost anti-aging drug absorption when compared to topical treatments. Hyaluronic acid (HA) has numerous applications in human medicine and the cosmetic industry [60].

Microneedling is a process that causes controlled micro-injuries to the skin, boosts collagen formation, and improves skin renewal. When paired with therapeutic chemicals given using MNs, this approach can improve skin restoration and cure diseases, including acne scars and stretch marks. Recent advancements include MN devices that provide growth factors or other regeneration agents to further improve skin results. Photoaging is extremely important for skin health and senescence. UV-vis irradiation disrupts the extracellular matrix microenvironment, degrades collagen, and induces oxidative stress. Traditional HA has a reduced potential to induce regeneration of collagen and is restricted due to its low macromolecule permeability, which limits the therapeutic benefits of photoaging [61].

The cosmetic industry has adopted MN technology in the creation of sophisticated skincare products. Home-use MN patches provide patients with improved delivery of moisturizing or brightening chemicals. These products are popular among people looking for noninvasive skincare solutions since they are both convenient and effective. Roussel et al. and colleagues found that inserting BIS-PNIPAm, a crosslinked polymer version, with dissolving MN patches improved mechanical qualities and resulted in a lower MN height decrease of around 10%. MNs made from PNIPAm alone lacked mechanical strength, necessitating the addition of polymeric excipients such as PVA to improve characteristics. The inclusion of a thermoresponsive polymer did not significantly affect needle insertion characteristics ($p > 0.05$). All formulations were inserted to a similar depth of 600 μm into ex vivo skin. The needles were loaded with a model payload, 1,1′-dioctadecyl-3,3,3′,3′-tetramethylindodicarbocyanine perchlorate (DID), and the cargo deposition was tracked via multiphoton microscopy, which revealed a deposit at a depth of around 200 μm. Crosslinked-PNIPAm (Bis-PNIPAm) formulations showed significant dye deposition in the skin after 4 hours, regardless of the excipient matrix utilized. The absence of this phenomenon in non-crosslinked PNIPAm formulations suggests a deposit development in the Bis-PNIPAm MN formulation. This proof-of-concept study suggests that PNIPAm can be used to create dissolving MNs, which can then be used to deposit nanoparticles in the dermis for prolonged drug release [62]. Many dermatological uses of MNs are given in **Table 2.**

iv. Pain and localized therapy - MNs provide novel alternatives for localized therapy and pain control by exploiting their accuracy and minimum invasiveness. MNs can administer analgesics directly to the source of pain, giving focused relief while avoiding systemic adverse effects. This method is useful for problems such as chronic muscle pain or joint inflammation, where standard pain drugs may be ineffective or create undesirable side effects. Recent research has shown that MNs are effective in delivering local anesthetics for procedures like dental work and small surgery. For chronic illnesses that require continuous treatment, MNs can provide sustained-release formulations that eliminate the need for frequent injection. MNs can be utilized to administer hormone replacement therapy or other chronic drugs, thereby enhancing patient compliance and therapeutic effects [77].

The capacity to tailor medication release profiles to individual demands is a significant advantage of MN technology. One potential method to deal with chronic wounds that reduce damage and encourage healing is early detection followed by prompt treatment. With the recent development of several smart dressings, active intervention, and real-time wound state monitoring are now possible. Inadequate effectiveness of treatment arises from the current smart dressing's shortcomings, which include limited drug loading capacity and poor drug penetration into deeper wound dermal and subcutaneous tissues. To accomplish simultaneous diagnosis and in-time therapy for chronic wounds, a closed-loop smart dressing with MN integrated has been designed. To track wound impedance and obtain early diagnoses of chronic wounds, simple impedance-detecting electrodes are employed [78]. The MeID drug delivery micropump is immediately activated for in-time therapy based on the sensing data. A practical solution for feeding adequate drug fluid into deeper wound dermal/subcutaneous tissues has been developed using micropump electrodes when combined with a drug reservoir-coupled MN array. Compared to untreated

	Area of discussion	Methods	Outcome	Reference
1.	Applications of MNs to enhance the look of the skin	An overview of using MNs to improve the appearance of the skin	It is possible to improve the appearance of skin with MNs.	[40]
2.	Needle dermabrasion	investigation on needle dermabrasion	The procedure of needle dermabrasion is used to rejuvenate skin.	[41]
3.	Using a derma roller for microneedling as a method of collagen induction therapy	Study on derma roller-assisted microneedling	Derma roller microneedling is a successful method of collagen induction therapy.	[42]
4.	An overview of an automated microneedling device—a new tool for a dermatologist's toolbox	An examination of automated microneedling equipment	In dermatology, automated microneedling equipment is talked about as a useful tool.	[45]
5.	Skin needling as a therapy for acne scars	Clinical investigation on skin needling for scarring from acne	An efficient treatment for acne scars is skin needling.	[46]
6.	Microneedling: Realities and myths	Examine the microneedling article	Investigates the truth and fiction behind skin care procedures using microneedling.	[63]
7.	Development under the guidance of constant ionic currents	Research on ionic currents' ability to regulate development	Examines the possibility of employing consistent ionic currents to regulate growth.	[64]
8.	A different approach to treating wrinkles, scars, and loose skin is percutaneous collagen induction therapy.	An investigation on Percutaneous Collagen Induction Therapy	A different approach to treating wrinkles, scars, and loose skin is called percutaneous collagen induction therapy.	[65]
9.	An overview of the data from in vitro research, animal experiments, and clinical trials on electrical stimulation for wound healing	An overview of electrical stimulation for the healing of wounds	Demonstrates how electrical stimulation aids in the healing of wounds.	[66]
10.	Minimally invasive procedure to induce collagen through the skin v	An overview of percutaneous minimally invasive collagen induction	Highlights the advantages of percutaneous collagen induction, a minimally invasive method, for skin rejuvenation.	[67]
11.	Microneedling improves liposomal sepia melani transfollicular absorption and dilates the follicular infundibulum.	Investigation into follicular dilatation and microneedling	The follicular infundibulum dilates, and transfollicular absorption is improved by microneedling.	[68]
12.	Wound recovery: The skin's biology	Information about the healing of wounds	Gives information about the biology of wound healing.	[69]
13.	The stimulation of skin cell growth by MNs	Research on the growth of skin cells using MNs	MNs promote the growth of skin cells.	[70]

	Area of discussion	Methods	Outcome	Reference
14.	Using percutaneous collagen induction therapy as a substitute for traditional burn scar therapy	Research on burn scars and percutaneous collagen induction therapy	Considered as an alternate therapy for burn scars is percutaneous collagen induction therapy.	[71]
15.	The Series of dermarollers	Details regarding the dermaroller line	Information about the dermaroller microneedling series.	[72]
16.	Using a dermaroller for microneedling	Article about using a dermal roller for microneedling	Describes the use of a derma roller for microneedling.	[73]
17.	Scars and wrinkles	Clinical investigation on surgery without subcutaneous incisions	Subcision works well to remove wrinkles and depressed scars.	[74]
18.	Dermatology in prime: The use of microneedling in treatment	An overview of the uses of microneedling	Explains the many uses of microneedling in the field of dermatology.	[75]
19.	Collagen induction treatment with derma rollers	Dermaroller experimentation with collagen induction therapy	For skin improvement, collagen induction therapy using dermarollers is explored.	[76]

Table 2.
Dermatological use of MNs.

diabetic mice, MelD stimulates faster wound healing in treated animals by supplying sufficient growth factors to the wound and boosting medication access into deep tissue layers. Meanwhile, MelD promotes tissue development and nascent collagen deposition. Meld's improved drug storage dosage, improved drug penetration, and closed-loop operation enable the first successful attempt to ensure sufficient and efficient drug delivery by miniaturized all-in-one smart dressing, expanding the use of closed-loop chronic wound care from a laboratory demonstration on limited types of superficial wounds to a broader range of wound types. A study found that an ingestible device activated by an external magnet can effectively treat sick locations in the intestinal tract. The capsule is designed to travel through the GI system and deliver MNs to targeted regions. This ingestible technology has the potential to enhance drug treatment efficacy and tolerance, paving the way for more effective GI illness management strategies [79].

6.2 Diagnostic applications

The diagnostic potential of nanoengineered MNs is equally groundbreaking, providing novel approaches for disease detection and monitoring. Continuous glucose monitoring (CGM) is an important part of diabetes therapy, and MNs have considerably improved this technology using the reactive oxygen species mechanism as described in **Figure 2**. Traditional glucose monitoring requires frequent blood samples, which can be painful and inconvenient for patients. MNs provide a minimally invasive option by capturing interstitial fluid for glucose readings. This strategy increases patient comfort and reduces the necessity for finger pricking, which is especially beneficial for diabetics. Continuous glucose monitors are essential for managing diabetes, but their general use is limited due to intrusive sampling, signal drift, and frequent calibrations. MN sensors provide a minimally invasive platform for real-time monitoring of clinical parameters in interstitial fluid. This study presents a painless and flexible MN sensing patch made of a robust MNs foundation and a thin layer of fluorescent hydrogel sensor for accurate and continuous glucose monitoring. FRET-based hydrogel sensors are made by photopolymerizing acryloylated FRET pairs with glucose-specific phenylboronic acid. The improved hydrogel sensor can measure glucose with reversibility, good selectivity, and signal stability against photobleaching. The MNs base is made of poly(ethylene glycol diacrylate)-polyacrylamide hydrogel, making it easier to pierce the skin and extract biofluid [7].

MN-based glucose sensors give real-time glucose level information, allowing insulin therapy to be adjusted as needed. These sensors can be included in wearable devices that constantly monitor glucose levels and notify patients of probable hypoglycemia or hyperglycemic situations. The real-time nature of these sensors helps to maintain better glucose management and reduce the risk of problems. Detachable MN sensors for continuous glucose monitoring (CGM) have a high therapeutic impact since they enable access to enormous data sets for personalized treatment approaches [80]. MN glucose sensors have advanced with the introduction of flexible and biocompatible materials that improve sensor performance and durability. Sensor technology advancements have resulted in more accurate and dependable glucose measurements, which have improved diabetes care. Ongoing research is aimed at improving the sensitivity and specificity of these sensors, allowing for even more precise glucose monitoring. A powerful wearable H_2O_2 MN sensor with a Prussian blue (PB)/carbon nanotube (CNT) composite electrode was created, as well as a glucose MN sensor based on it [81].

MNs are making progress in the identification of illness biomarkers, providing a less invasive way to diagnose and monitor a variety of disorders. MNs loaded with particular antibodies or molecular probes can detect cancer indicators in interstitial fluid. This noninvasive technique allows for early cancer identification and disease progression tracking. MNs have been shown in studies to detect biomarkers associated with a variety of malignancies, including breast, prostate, and colorectal. This capability enables timely intervention and individualized treatment solutions. There are numerous ways for early tumor detection, including identifying circulating tumor DNA, detecting circulating tumor cells, and imaging with tumor-targeting contrast agents. However, these assays are time-consuming and may cause discomfort for the patient during the biopsy collection procedure. We present a simple approach for early tumor diagnosis that involves collecting exosomes from interstitial fluid (ISF) with hydrogel MNs (MNs). The hydrogel MNs stretch in the skin to absorb the ISF, and tumor exosomes in the ISF bind to glypican-1 antibodies within the MN hydrogel. Exosomes are separated from the ISF and analyzed for tumor-related biomarkers when the hydrogel on the MNs is removed. Finally, colon cancer can be detected by ELISA in colorectal cancer-induced model mice. This noninvasive hydrogel MN method for obtaining exosome samples would be very useful in early cancer diagnosis [82]. MNs can also be employed to detect infections by capturing microbial or viral biomarkers. For example, MNs functionalized with probes for specific pathogens can provide rapid diagnostic results, facilitating early treatment and containment of infectious diseases. Recent advancements include the development of MNs for detecting biomarkers associated with emerging infectious

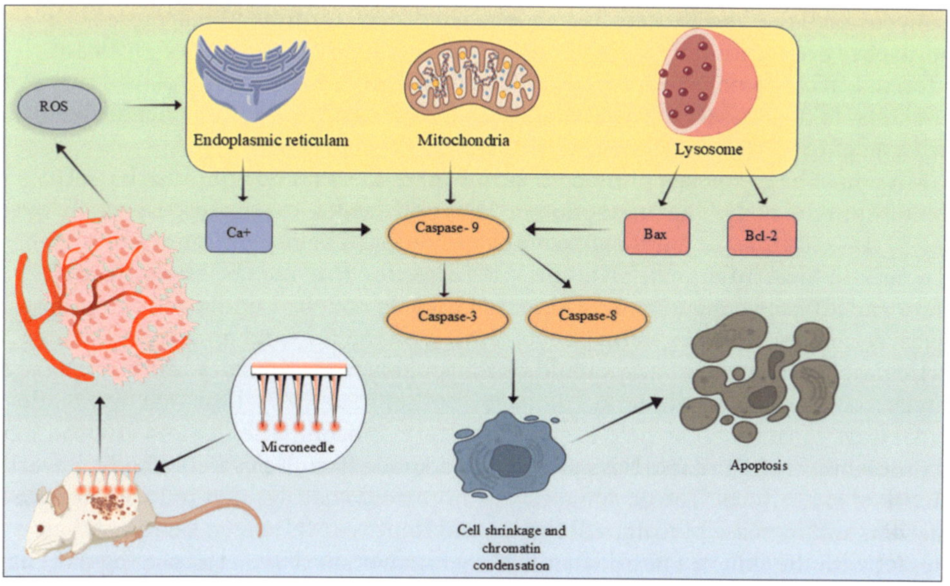

Figure 3.
MNs can enhance drug delivery by penetrating the skin, creating microchannels that allow for targeted release. This process can induce the production of Reactive oxygen species (ROS), which plays a role in signaling and can contribute to therapeutic effects, especially in treatments like cancer therapy.

diseases, such as COVID-19. A polymeric MNs coupled electrochemical sensor array (MNESA) was used by the researchers to monitor kidney biomarkers in the skin interstitial fluid (ISF) in real time, with minimal invasiveness and self-administration [83]. The combination of MNs with microfluidic technologies has improved biomarker detection and analysis. These sophisticated systems have higher sensitivity and specificity for identifying a wide range of biomarkers, making them useful for both research and clinical diagnosis. Innovations in NM coatings and sensor technology are propelling this sector forward. MNs can enhance drug delivery by penetrating the skin, creating microchannels that allow for targeted release. This process can induce the production of Reactive oxygen species (ROS), which plays a role in signaling and can contribute to therapeutic effects, especially in treatments like cancer therapy, as explained in **Figure 3.**

7. Challenges and future directions

Scaling up the manufacturing of MNs necessitates complicated fabrication techniques and quality control procedures. Maintaining uniformity and reproducibility in large-scale manufacturing presents a substantial challenge. Manufacturing advancements, including roll-to-roll processing and injection molding, are being investigated to make large-scale production more practical. Research into cost-effective and scalable fabrication methods is vital for the broad adoption of MN technology. A unique manufacturing procedure for creating MN arrays has been developed and tested. The prototype can manufacture 14-14 MN arrays and can be scaled up, making it suitable for transitioning from lab to industry and commercialization. To create silicone MN molds using injection molding, metal master templates must be custom-designed. This innovative approach was compared to centrifugation, a conventional method for creating aqueous hydrogel-forming MN arrays. Both approaches produced MN arrays of equivalent quality, indicating no significant difference in outcomes. Both types of MN arrays can be successfully placed into skin simulants. In both cases, the insertion depth was roughly 70% of the needle length, with a height reduction of about 3% [84].

MNs must be composed of biocompatible materials that do not cause harmful responses in the body. The interaction of MNs with biological tissues, especially over long periods of time, requires extensive examination. The risk of immunological responses or local inflammation at the MN's insertion site must be assessed. MNs' safety and efficacy depend on ensuring that they do not elicit undesired immunological responses. The long-term effects of MNs on the skin and underlying tissues, particularly with frequent use, should be thoroughly investigated. Chronic exposure or recurrent use may result in skin damage or other issues [85]. Research into biodegradable MN materials can help to solve long-term biocompatibility and environmental problems. Biodegradable MNs dissolve or degrade harmlessly in the body, lowering the risk of side effects. The development of improved coatings that reduce immune reactions and increase biocompatibility would improve MN safety. Coatings that interact with the skin in a non-inflammatory manner are critical to assuring patient comfort and safety. Extensive preclinical and clinical experiments are required to evaluate the long-term safety and biocompatibility of MNs. Detailed investigations on their effects on various skin types and demographics will help us better understand their safety profile [86].

The integration of nanotechnology into medical equipment complicates regulatory authorization. Regulations governing the usage of NMs and their interactions with the human body are constantly changing. Gaining regulatory approval for MN-based devices requires extensive testing and documentation to demonstrate safety, efficacy, and quality. The procedure can be time-consuming and expensive [25]. Engaging with regulatory bodies early in the development phase can assist in resolving potential issues and speeding up the approval process. Collaborative efforts can result in clearer guidelines and faster regulatory processes. Establishing consistent testing techniques for MN products will make regulatory assessments go more smoothly and assure product uniformity. It is critical for worldwide deployment to navigate different countries' regulatory constraints. Harmonizing international rules and developing a single approach can help to accelerate the global adoption of MN technologies [85].

8. Regulatory requirements

Considering that MN systems are a relatively new technology in the pharmaceutical industry and that, as previously mentioned, there are four different types of MN systems that are manufactured using a variety of technologies, industry, and researchers need standardized guidelines for the use of established techniques for production, evaluation, test criteria for approval, and quality control. Consequently, the FDA released "Regulatory Considerations for Microneedling Devices" and "Scientific Considerations for MN Products" in 2017 to support the development of MNs as medical devices in accordance with Section 201 (h) of the Federal Food, Drug, and Cosmetic Act [87].

MNs are medical devices designed to treat or track a certain ailment. MNs are classified as class II devices under 21 CFR 878.4430 and come with a variety of sharp

Clinical trial	Disease/disorder	Analyte	Outcome
NCT02682056	Pediatric diabetes	Glucose	Comparative analysis of the effectiveness of intravenous catheters versus MN patches over lancets for the monitoring of blood glucose in children with diabetes.
NCT05546229	Opioid abuse disorders	Buprenorphine	Use of MNs to examine the detectability of popular drugs used to treat opioid use disorders and their metabolites in dISF.
NCT03847610	Resistance to antibiotics	Beta-lactam	An assessment of the effectiveness of an MN electrochemical biosensor for benzylpenicillin level monitoring in relation to microdialysis and blood collection techniques.
NCT04238611	Thresholds for anaerobic metabolism	Lactate	Validation of an MN-based instrument for continuous lactate monitoring during physical activity.
NCT01908530	Type 1 diabetes	Glucose	An electrochemical microprobe array with entrapped glucose oxidase for continuous glucose monitoring is evaluated for safety and effectiveness.
NCT05922176	Opioid abuse disorders	Methadone	Detectability evaluation of popular drugs used to treat opioid use disorders and their metabolites in dISF using MNs.
NCT05998876	Opioid abuse disorder	methadone	Using differential pulse voltammetry integrated on an MN electrode array, methadone detection in ISF and continuous monitoring of methadone adherence.

Table 3.
Clinical trial of diagnostic MNs.

ends, similar to hypodermic needles. These goods fall into one of two categories: combination products, which are overseen by the US FDA's CBER (Center for Biological Evaluation and Research) or CDER (Center for Drug Evaluation and Research) divisions, or medical devices, which are governed by the CDRH (Center for Devices and Radiological Health). The labeling for these kinds of devices must contain information on the device's components, technical specifications (such as needle geometry and insertion depth), recommended course of treatment, disposal guidelines, processing instructions for reusable items, and expiration date. Comprehensive research on metabolism and elimination pathways is undoubtedly needed by regulatory bodies, which could delay commercialization. Authorities require that MN systems be sterile since, in contrast to conventional transdermal and topical drug delivery systems, they come into contact with live skin cells [28]. Clinical trial of diagnostic MNs given in **Table 3.**

9. Future directions

Future studies could focus on creating MNs with several functions, such as diagnostic and therapeutic capabilities. MNs that can detect biomarkers as well as administer medications would be extremely useful in theragnostic applications. The use of smart technologies, such as sensors and microelectronic components, may allow MNs to adapt to physiological changes or environmental variables. Smart MNs could regulate medicine release rates or deliver real-time diagnostic information dependent on the patient's state. Expanding the use of MNs to treat chronic diseases other than diabetes and cancer is a critical area of development. MNs could be used to treat cardiovascular illness, neurological diseases, and respiratory ailments, providing long-term drug delivery or monitoring options. MNs can be further improved to support personalized medicine techniques, which adjust diagnosis and treatment based on individual genetic, metabolic, or physiological characteristics. Personalized MN devices may increase the precision and effectiveness of healthcare interventions. Integrating MNs with wearable technologies, such as smart patches or health monitoring systems, may increase their usefulness in continuous health monitoring and illness management. Wearable devices using MNs might monitor vital signs, glucose levels, and other health metrics in real time. MN-based diagnostic technologies could be integrated into telemedicine platforms to provide remote health monitoring and data collection. This connection would allow healthcare providers to better manage patient care and intervene quickly when needed. Creating novel biocompatible polymers and nanocomposites for MNs will improve their performance and safety. Research into materials with higher mechanical strength, longevity, and biocompatibility will improve the overall effectiveness of MN devices. Integrating self-healing materials into MNs may increase their durability and lifetime. Self-healing materials could fix slight damage to MNs while in use, assuring consistent performance and decreasing the need for frequent replacements.

10. Conclusion

Nanoengineered MNs are on the verge of transforming both therapeutic and diagnostic uses in modern medication. Their versatility in delivering medications, vaccines, and therapeutic agents, combined with the promise of increased diagnostic capabilities, makes them a critical technology for the future of healthcare. Despite manufacturing, biocompatibility, and regulatory approval hurdles, current research and innovation show promise in overcoming these barriers and realizing MN's full potential. The future of MN technology is to improve functionalization, increase clinical application, integrate with digital health technologies, and advance material science. By addressing present obstacles and following these future paths, MNs will help to progress the field of theragnostic, providing more effective, tailored, and accessible healthcare options. As technology advances, nanoengineered MNs have the potential to significantly improve patient care and shape the future of medicine.

Abbreviation

HA	hyaluronic acid
MN	microneedle
NM	nanomaterial
sdMN	self-dissolving MNs

DOI: http://dx.doi.org/10.5772/intechopen.1009262

Author details

Mansi Singh and Rahul Shukla*
Department of Pharmaceutics, National Institute of Pharmaceutical Education and Research-Raebareli, Lucknow, UP, India

*Address all correspondence to: rahulshuklapharm@gmail.com; rahul.shukla@niperraebareli.edu.in

References

[1] Amani H, Shahbazi MA, Damico C, Fontana F, Abbaszadeh S, Santos HA. Microneedles for painless transdermal immunotherapeutic applications. Journal of Controlled Release. 2021;**330**:185-217

[2] Haridass IN, Wei JCJ, Mohammed YH, Crichton ML, Anderson CD, Henricson J, et al. Cellular metabolism and pore lifetime of human skin following microprojection array mediation. Journal of Controlled Release. 2019;**306**:59-68

[3] Chen X, Xiao H, Zhao Q, Xu X, Cen Y, Xiao D. Research hotspot and trend of microneedles in biomedical field: A bibliometric analysis from 2011 to 2020. Burns. 2022;**48**(4):959-972

[4] Deng J, Wang Z, Zhou Z, Yu W, Li X, Song Z, et al. Transdermal delivery of Fluoropolymer-modified microneedle vaccines against rabies elicits potent humoral immunity. Chemical Engineering Journal. 2023;**474**:145496

[5] Yang G, Xu W, Xu B, Yang Y, Li P, Yu A, et al. Two decades' advancements and research trends in needle-type sensor technology: A scientometric analysis. Heliyon. 2024;**10**(6):e27399

[6] Park K. Collective progress in drug delivery. Journal of Controlled Release. 2019;**300**:197-199

[7] Hu Y, Pan Z, De Bock M, Tan TX, Wang Y, Shi Y, et al. A wearable microneedle patch incorporating reversible FRET-based hydrogel sensors for continuous glucose monitoring. Biosensors & Bioelectronics. 2024;**262**:116542

[8] Donadei A, Kraan H, Ophorst O, Flynn O, O'Mahony C, Soema PC, et al. Skin delivery of trivalent Sabin inactivated poliovirus vaccine using dissolvable microneedle patches induces neutralizing antibodies. Journal of Controlled Release. 2019;**311-312**:96-103

[9] Wang W, Zhong Z, Peng S, Fu J, Chen M, Lang T, et al. "All-in-one" metal polyphenol network nanocapsules integrated microneedle patches for lipophagy fueled ferroptosis-mediated multimodal therapy. Journal of Controlled Release. 2024;**373**:599-616

[10] Yan Q, Weng J, Shen S, Wang Y, Fang M, Zheng G, et al. Finite element analysis for biodegradable dissolving microneedle materials on skin puncture and mechanical performance evaluation. Polymers (Basel). 2021;**13**(18):3043

[11] Yao Z, Xue T, Xiong H, Cai C, Liu X, Wu F, et al. Promotion of collagen deposition during skin healing through Smad3/mTOR pathway by parathyroid hormone-loaded microneedle. Materials Science and Engineering: C. 2021;**119**:111446

[12] Park Y, Kim KS, Chung M, Sung JH, Kim B. Fabrication and characterization of dissolving microneedle arrays for improving skin permeability of cosmetic ingredients. Journal of Industrial and Engineering Chemistry. 2016;**39**:121-126

[13] Tan G, Ioannou N, Mathew E, Tagalakis AD, Lamprou DA, Yu-Wai-Man C. 3D printing in ophthalmology: From medical implants to personalised medicine. International Journal of Pharmaceutics. 2022;**625**:122094

[14] Kumar S, Shukla R. Advancements in microneedle technology: Current status and next-generation innovations. Journal of Microencapsulation. 2024;**41**(8):782-803

[15] Krieger KJ, Bertollo N, Dangol M, Sheridan JT, Lowery MM, O'Cearbhaill ED. Simple and customizable method for fabrication of high-aspect ratio microneedle molds using low-cost 3D printing. Microsystems and Nanoengineering. 2019;**5**(1):42

[16] Liu GS, Kong Y, Wang Y, Luo Y, Fan X, Xie X, et al. Microneedles for transdermal diagnostics: Recent advances and new horizons. Biomaterials. 2020;**232**:119740

[17] Economidou SN, Douroumis D. 3D printing as a transformative tool for microneedle systems: Recent advances, manufacturing considerations and market potential. Advanced Drug Delivery Reviews. 2021;**173**:60-69

[18] Li R, Zhang L, Jiang X, Li L, Wu S, Yuan X, et al. 3D-printed microneedle arrays for drug delivery. Journal of Controlled Release. 2022;**350**:933-948

[19] Yang J, Liu X, Fu Y, Song Y. Recent advances of microneedles for biomedical applications: Drug delivery and beyond. Acta Pharmaceutica Sinica B. 2019;**9**(3):469-483

[20] Kang L, Kochhar C, Zou S. Protein encapsulation in polymeric microneedles by photolithography. International Journal of Nanomedicine. 2012;**3143**

[21] Dardano P, Caliò A, Di Palma V, Bevilacqua M, Di Matteo A, De Stefano L. A photolithographic approach to polymeric microneedles Array fabrication. Materials. 2015;**8**(12):8661-8673

[22] Kathuria H, Kang K, Cai J, Kang L. Rapid microneedle fabrication by heating and photolithography. International Journal of Pharmaceutics. 2020;**575**:118992

[23] Li Y, Zhang H, Yang R, Laffitte Y, Schmill U, Hu W, et al. Fabrication of sharp silicon hollow microneedles by deep-reactive ion etching towards minimally invasive diagnostics. Microsystems and Nanoengineering. 2019;**5**(1):41

[24] Bolton CJW, Howells O, Blayney GJ, Eng PF, Birchall JC, Gualeni B, et al. Hollow silicon microneedle fabrication using advanced plasma etch technologies for applications in transdermal drug delivery. Lab on a Chip. 2020;**20**(15):2788-2795

[25] Singh M, Shukla R. Leveraging nanoengineered microneedle-augmented drug delivery in oncological intervention. Particle and Particle Systems Characterization. 2024

[26] Donnelly RF, Singh TRR, Garland MJ, Migalska K, Majithiya R, McCrudden CM, et al. Hydrogel-forming microneedle arrays for enhanced transdermal drug delivery. Advanced Functional Materials. 2012;**22**(23):4879-4890

[27] Shukla S, Mamale KB, Arya RKK, Kaundal RK, Shukla R. Therapeutic potential of microneedles based delivery systems for the management of atopic dermatitis. Journal of Drug Delivery Science and Technology. 2023;**84**:104493

[28] Larrañeta E, Lutton REM, Woolfson AD, Donnelly RF. Microneedle arrays as transdermal and intradermal drug delivery systems: Materials science, manufacture and commercial development. Materials Science and Engineering: R: Reports. 2016;**104**:1-32

[29] Zhong G, Liu Q, Wang Q, Qiu H, Li H, Xu T. Fully integrated microneedle biosensor array for wearable multiplexed fitness biomarkers monitoring.

Biosensors and Bioelectronics. 2024;**265**:116697

[30] Forvi E, Bedoni M, Carabalona R, Soncini M, Mazzoleni P, Rizzo F, et al. Preliminary technological assessment of microneedles-based dry electrodes for biopotential monitoring in clinical examinations. Sensors and Actuators A: Physical. 2012;**180**:177-186

[31] Tiwari N, Aggarwal G, Jain GK, Mittal G. Multi-drug loaded microneedles for emergency treatment of snakebite envenomation. Medical Hypotheses. 2022;**165**:110908

[32] Wu D, Wu X, Luan Q, Tang Q, Fan L, Shou X, et al. Dynamic hydrogel-integrated microneedle patch with extracellular vesicles encapsulation for wound healing. Chemical Engineering Journal. 2024;**493**:152252

[33] Lin Y, Chen Y, Deng R, Qin H, Li N, Qin Y, et al. Delivery of neutrophil membrane encapsulated non-steroidal anti-inflammatory drugs by degradable biopolymer microneedle patch for rheumatoid arthritis therapy. Nano Today. 2023;**49**:101791

[34] Arora P, Shukla R. Microneedles along with conventional therapies: An in-depth observational review in alopecia areata treatment. Journal of Drug Delivery Science and Technology. 2024;**95**:105627

[35] Zhang X, Chen H, Song T, Wang J, Zhao Y. Controllable histotomy based on hierarchical magnetic microneedle array robots. Engineering. 2024;**42**

[36] Ito S, Hirobe S, Yamashita R, Sugiyama A, Takeuchi H, Eguchi R, et al. Analysis of immune response induction mechanisms implicating the dose-sparing effect of transcutaneous immunization using a self-dissolving microneedle patch. Vaccine. 2022;**40**(6):862-872

[37] Kim JY, Han MR, Kim YH, Shin SW, Nam SY, Park JH. Tip-loaded dissolving microneedles for transdermal delivery of donepezil hydrochloride for treatment of Alzheimer's disease. European Journal of Pharmaceutics and Biopharmaceutics. 2016;**105**:148-155

[38] Danne T, Heinemann L, Bolinder J. New insulins, biosimilars, and insulin therapy. Diabetes Technology and Therapeutics. 2016;**18**(S1):S-43-S-55

[39] Cao J, Zhang N, Wang Z, Su J, Yang J, Han J, et al. Microneedle-assisted transdermal delivery of etanercept for rheumatoid arthritis treatment. Pharmaceutics. 2019;**11**(5):235

[40] Dangol M, Kim S, Li CG, Fakhraei Lahiji S, Jang M, Ma Y, et al. Anti-obesity effect of a novel caffeine-loaded dissolving microneedle patch in high-fat diet-induced obese C57BL/6J mice. Journal of Controlled Release. 2017;**265**:41-47

[41] Cao J, Su J, An M, Yang Y, Zhang Y, Zuo J, et al. Novel DEK-targeting aptamer delivered by a hydrogel microneedle attenuates collagen-induced arthritis. Molecular Pharmaceutics. 2021;**18**(1):305-316

[42] Zhang Y, Liu Q, Yu J, Yu S, Wang J, Qiang L, et al. Locally induced adipose tissue browning by microneedle patch for obesity treatment. ACS Nano. 2017;**11**(9):9223-9230

[43] Li B, Lu G, Liu W, Liao L, Ban J, Lu Z. Formulation and evaluation of PLGA nanoparticulate-based microneedle system for potential treatment of neurological diseases. International Journal of Nanomedicine. 2023;**18**:3745-3760

[44] Tan S, Wang Y, Wei X, Xiao X, Gao L. Microneedle-mediated drug

delivery for neurological diseases. International Journal of Pharmaceutics. 2024;**661**:124400

[45] Jiang J, Gill HS, Ghate D, McCarey BE, Patel SR, Edelhauser HF, et al. Coated microneedles for drug delivery to the eye. Investigative Opthalmology and Visual Science. 2007;**48**(9):4038

[46] Martanto W, Moore JS, Kashlan O, Kamath R, Wang PM, O'Neal JM, et al. Microinfusion using hollow microneedles. Pharmaceutical Research. 2006;**23**(1):104-113

[47] Yenkoidiok-Douti L, Barillas-Mury C, Jewell CM. Design of dissolvable microneedles for delivery of a Pfs47-based malaria transmission-blocking vaccine. ACS Biomaterials Science and Engineering. 2021;7(5):1854-1862

[48] Matsuo K, Hirobe S, Yokota Y, Ayabe Y, Seto M, Quan YS, et al. Transcutaneous immunization using a dissolving microneedle array protects against tetanus, diphtheria, malaria, and influenza. Journal of Controlled Release. 2012;**160**(3):495-501

[49] Carey JB, Pearson FE, Vrdoljak A, McGrath MG, Crean AM, Walsh PT, et al. Microneedle array design determines the induction of protective memory CD8+ T cell responses induced by a recombinant live malaria vaccine in mice. PLoS One. 2011;**6**(7):e22442

[50] Jamaledin R, Yiu CKY, Zare EN, Niu L, Vecchione R, Chen G, et al. Advances in antimicrobial microneedle patches for combating infections. Advanced Materials. 2020;**32**(33)

[51] Gadziński P, Froelich A, Wojtyłko M, Białek A, Krysztofiak J, Osmałek T. Microneedle-based ocular drug delivery systems – Recent advances and challenges. Beilstein Journal of Nanotechnology. 2022;**13**:1167-1184

[52] Phoka T, Thanuthanakhun N, Visitchanakun P, Dueanphen N, Wanichwecharungruang N, Leelahavanichkul A, et al. Detachable-dissolvable-microneedle as a potent subunit vaccine delivery device that requires no cold-chain. Vaccine X. 2023;**15**:100398

[53] Nguyen TT, Van Vo G. Microneedle-mediated vaccine delivery. In: Design and Applications of Microneedles in Drug Delivery and Therapeutics. Jamia Hamdard, New Delhi, India: Department of Pharmaceutics, School of Pharmaceutical Education and Research; 2024. pp. 433-448

[54] Qiu H, Gong L, Slezak P, He S, Lu F, Yu K, et al. Magnetic-navigable silk fibroin microneedles for oral drug delivery: Ensuring long-lasting helicobacter pylori eradication and rapid hemostasis in the stomach. International Journal of Biological Macromolecules. 2024;**275**:133584

[55] Phoka T, Wanichwecharungruang N, Dueanphen N, Thanuthanakhun N, Kietdumrongwong P, Leelahavanichkul A, et al. Converting short-acting insulin into thermo-stable longer-acting insulin using multi-layer detachable microneedles. Journal of Pharmaceutical Sciences. 2024;**113**

[56] Huang J, Yao Z, Li B, Ping Y. Targeted delivery of PROTAC-based prodrug activated by bond-cleavage bioorthogonal chemistry for microneedle-assisted cancer therapy. Journal of Controlled Release. 2023;**361**:270-279

[57] Castilla-Casadiego DA, Carlton H, Gonzalez-Nino D, Miranda-Muñoz KA, Daneshpour R, Huitink D, et al. Design,

characterization, and modeling of a chitosan microneedle patch for transdermal delivery of meloxicam as a pain management strategy for use in cattle. Materials Science and Engineering: C. 2021;**118**:111544

[58] Ramadon D, Karn PR, Anjani QK, Kim MH, Cho DY, Hwang H, et al. Development of ropivacaine hydrochloride-loaded dissolving microneedles as a local anesthetic agent: A proof-of-concept. International Journal of Pharmaceutics. 2024;**660**:124347

[59] Glover K, Mishra D, Gade S, Vora LK, Wu Y, Paredes AJ, et al. Microneedles for advanced ocular drug delivery. Advanced Drug Delivery Reviews. 2023;**201**:115082

[60] Zhang JN, Chen BZ, Ashfaq M, Zhang XP, Guo XD. Development of a BDDE-crosslinked hyaluronic acid based microneedles patch as a dermal filler for anti-ageing treatment. Journal of Industrial and Engineering Chemistry. 2018;**65**:363-369

[61] Tang Z, Liu Z, Zhang Y, Luo S, Xu Y, Ren L. Functional hyaluronic acid microneedles for skin photoaging based on collagen induction and oxidative stress regulation strategies. International Journal of Biological Macromolecules. 2024;**277**:134080

[62] Roussel S, Udabe J, Bin Sabri A, Calderón M, Donnelly R. Leveraging novel innovative thermoresponsive polymers in microneedles for targeted intradermal deposition. International Journal of Pharmaceutics. 2024;**652**:123847

[63] Chang H, Zheng M, Yu X, Than A, Seeni RZ, Kang R, et al. A swellable microneedle patch to rapidly extract skin interstitial fluid for timely metabolic analysis. Advanced Materials. 2017;**29**(37)

[64] Shende P, Salunke M. Transepidermal microneedles for co-administration of folic acid with methotrexate in the treatment of rheumatoid arthritis. Biomedical Physics and Engineering Express. 2019;**5**(2):025023

[65] Lee JW, Park JH, Prausnitz MR. Dissolving microneedles for transdermal drug delivery. Biomaterials. 2008;**29**(13):2113-2124

[66] Goh GD, Sing SL, Yeong WY. A review on machine learning in 3D printing: Applications, potential, and challenges. Artificial Intelligence Review. 2021;**54**(1):63-94

[67] Lau S, Fei J, Liu H, Chen W, Liu R. Multilayered pyramidal dissolving microneedle patches with flexible pedestals for improving effective drug delivery. Journal of Controlled Release. 2017;**265**:113-119

[68] Jung J, Dos Santos e Lucato SL. A CDM-based binary model for the progressive damage prediction of sic/sic ceramic matrix composites under tension loading. International Journal for Multiscale Computational Engineering. 2021;**19**(5):1-15

[69] Kim YC, Park JH, Prausnitz MR. Microneedles for drug and vaccine delivery. Advanced Drug Delivery Reviews. 2012;**64**(14):1547-1568

[70] Liu S, Jin M, Shu QY, Kamiyama F, Kusamori K, Katsumi H, et al. Transdermal delivery of relatively high molecular weight drugs using novel self-dissolving microneedle arrays fabricated from hyaluronic acid and their characteristics and safety after application to the skin. European Journal of Pharmaceutics and Biopharmaceutics. 2014;**86**(2):267-276

[71] Aust MC, Knobloch K, Reimers K, Redeker J, Ipaktchi R, Altintas MA, et al.

Percutaneous collagen induction therapy: An alternative treatment for burn scars. Burns. 2010;**36**(6):836-843

[72] Tiller W. In memoriam Wolfgang Boehm. Computer-Aided Design and Applications. 2018;**15**(6):779-779

[73] Kumar A, Naguib YW, Shi Y, chun, Cui Z. A method to improve the efficacy of topical eflornithine hydrochloride cream. Drug Delivery. 2014;**23**(5):1-7

[74] Orentreich DS, Orentreich N. Subcutaneous incisionless (subcision) surgery for the correction of depressed scars and wrinkles. Dermatologic Surgery. 1995;**21**(6):543-549

[75] Kim M, Yang H, Kim H, Jung H, Jung H. Novel cosmetic patches for wrinkle improvement: Retinyl retinoate- and ascorbic acid-loaded dissolving microneedles. International Journal of Cosmetic Science. 2014;**36**(3):207-212

[76] Prausnitz MR, Mikszta JA, Cormier M, Andrianov AK. Microneedle-Based Vaccines. Shivaprasad Gadag, Manipal, Karnataka, India: Department of Pharmaceutics, Manipal College of Pharmaceutical Sciences, Manipal Academy of Higher Education; 2009. pp. 369-393

[77] Gadag S, Narayan R, Nayak AS, Catalina Ardila D, Sant S, Nayak Y, et al. Development and preclinical evaluation of microneedle-assisted resveratrol loaded nanostructured lipid carriers for localized delivery to breast cancer therapy. International Journal of Pharmaceutics. 2021;**606**:120877

[78] Jha A, Kumar M, Goswami P, Manjit M, Bharti K, Koch B, et al. Hyaluronic acid-oleylamine and chitosan-oleic acid conjugate-based hybrid nanoparticle delivery via. Dissolving microneedles for enhanced treatment efficacy in localized breast cancer. Biomaterials. Advances. 2024;**160**:213865

[79] Levy JA, Straker MA, Stine JM, Beardslee LA, Ghodssi R. Magnetically triggered ingestible capsule for localized microneedle drug delivery. Device. 2024;**100438**

[80] Li L, Zhou Y, Sun C, Zhou Z, Zhang J, Xu Y, et al. Fully integrated wearable microneedle biosensing platform for wide-range and real-time continuous glucose monitoring. Acta Biomaterialia. 2024;**175**:199-213

[81] Zhu J, Wang L, Xu S, Peng L, Gao Z, Liu S, et al. A high-performance wearable microneedle sensor based on a prussian blue-carbon nanotube composite electrode for the detection of hydrogen peroxide and glucose. Sensors and Actuators B: Chemical. 2024;**419**:136436

[82] Park W, Maeng SW, Mok JW, Choi M, Cha HJ, Joo CK, et al. Hydrogel microneedles extracting exosomes for early detection of colorectal cancer. Biomacromolecules. 2023;**24**(3):1445-1452

[83] Zheng L, Zhu D, Xiao Y, Zheng X, Chen P. Microneedle coupled epidermal sensor for multiplexed electrochemical detection of kidney disease biomarkers. Biosensors and Bioelectronics. 2023;**237**:115506

[84] Lutton REM, Larrañeta E, Kearney MC, Boyd P, Woolfson AD, Donnelly RF. A novel scalable manufacturing process for the production of hydrogel-forming microneedle arrays. International Journal of Pharmaceutics. 2015;**494**(1):417-429

[85] Wendong Y, Xingxing Y, Xianze X, Qiaomei F, Yujun S, Shanshan Z, et al.

Nanoformulation-assisted microneedle transdermal drug delivery system: An innovative platform enhancing rheumatoid arthritis treatment. Biomedicine and Pharmacotherapy. 2024;**178**:117219

[86] Wu C, Yu Q, Huang C, Li F, Zhang L, Zhu D. Microneedles as transdermal drug delivery system for enhancing skin disease treatment. Acta Pharmaceutica Sinica B. 2024;**14**

[87] Babity S, Roohnikan M, Brambilla D. Advances in the Design of Transdermal Microneedles for diagnostic and monitoring applications. Small. 2018;**14**(49)

Section 2

Mechnastic Innovation of Advanced Formulation

Chapter 4

Liposomal Technology in Drug Formulations: Enhancing Therapeutic Efficacy and Safety

Vaibhavi Patel and Pranav Y. Dave

Abstract

Liposomes are vesicular structures made of lipid bilayers that naturally develop when phospholipids scatter in water. These small vesicles included an aqueous core within a membrane made of lipid bilayers. Novel Drug Delivery Systems (NDDS) are intended to release medications at a controlled rate dependent on the body's needs during therapy while targeting specific locations of action. Liposomes, which are spherical structures made up of phospholipid bilayers, have gained popularity in therapeutic formulations due to their ability to encapsulate both hydrophilic and hydrophobic medicines. This dual encapsulation capability improves the therapeutic efficacy and safety of many medicines. Liposomes are ideal for targeted drug delivery due to their biocompatibility, biodegradability, and non-immunogenic qualities, which reduce systemic side effects and improve bioavailability. Recent advances in liposomal technology have resulted in formulations being employed in a variety of sectors, including cancer therapy, infectious disorders, and vaccine administration. This review examines the structural properties, preparation methodologies, and therapeutic applications of liposomes, emphasising their potential to change drug delivery systems. This chapter emphasises the crucial importance of liposomes in modern pharmaceutical sciences and their bright future in personalised medicine by examining current research and clinical applications.

Keywords: liposome, phospholipid structure, hydrophilic and hydrophobic drugs, formulation, drug delivery

1. Introduction

Liposomes represent spherical vesicles, comprising one or more phospholipid bilayers first described in the 1960s by the British haematologist Alec D. Bang ham with the ability to encapsulate both hydrophilic and lipophilic drugs. In 1965, researchers presented the first description of swelling phospholipid systems. Within a few years, a variety of enclosed phospholipid bilayer structures made up of single bilayers, dubbed 'bangosomes' and then 'liposomes', were described. Early pioneers such as Gregoriadis and Perrie demonstrated that liposomes can entrap pharmaceuticals and be employed as drug delivery devices [1]. Due to this structure, liposomes have become a really effective drug delivery system through which they improve the therapeutic index of drugs by enhancing their bioavailability, prolonging circulation time, and reducing toxicity. Since these vesicles tend to imitate cell membranes, they are biocompatible and are, therefore, capable of delivering drugs to the site of their target either through passive or active targeting mechanisms. This drastically reduces side effects and increases the therapeutic value of the drugs being used [2].

Therefore, liposomes have been employed in many fields of medical science, ranging from oncology to infectious diseases and gene therapy. The ability of liposomes to encapsulate drugs either within their aqueous core or within their lipid bilayer enables them to protect labile drugs from degradation and allows for controlled release, hence making them an attractive vehicle for a number of therapeutic agents [3]. More recent advances in liposomal technology have improved circulation time in the bloodstream, through processes such as pegylation, offering new opportunities in both precision medicine and personalised therapies [4]. Liposomes are composed of amphiphilic phospholipids with a hydrophilic head and a hydrophobic tail, which allows them to seal themselves in aquatic environments. In recent years, major research has concentrated on the delivery of antibiotics [5, 6], genes [7, 8], antifungals [9, 10], anti-inflammatory [11, 12], and anticancer drugs [13, 14], which are also used in many pharmacological, biological, and medical applications.

2. Structure of liposome

The primary structural components of liposomes are phospholipids and cholesterol. The lipid bilayer is made up of phospholipids with a hydrophilic head and a hydrophobic tail group. The head attracts water, while the tail, which is formed of a long hydrocarbon chain, repels water. Phospholipids, the primary component of liposomes, can easily merge with skin lipids, enhancing medication penetration and localisation in the skin layers. The cholesterol absorbed into the lipid membrane increases the stability of liposomes while also reducing membrane permeability. As bilayer structures, liposomes in aqueous solution can encapsulate hydrophilic compounds in the aqueous compartment while hydrophobic substances can be accommodated in the lipid phase (**Figure 1**) [15].

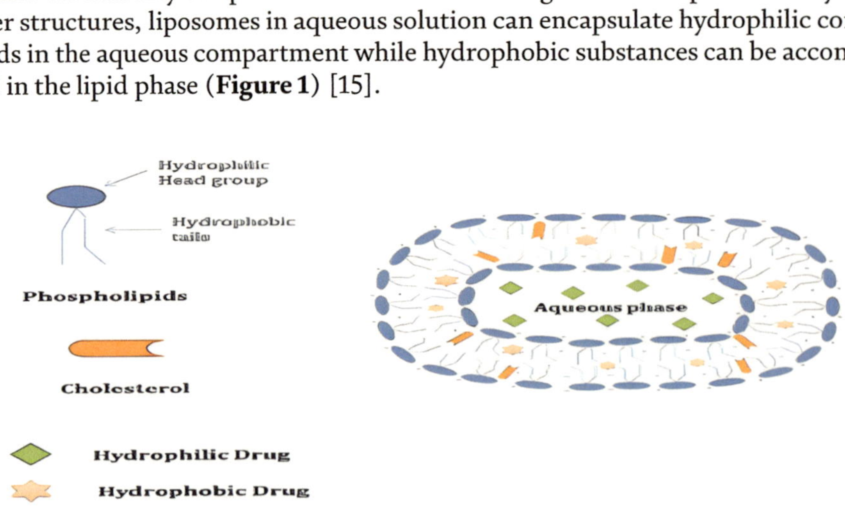

Figure 1.
Structure of conventional liposome encapsulating hydrophilic & hydrophobic drugs.

3. The way that liposomes work

A liposome is an aqueous solution surrounded by a hydrophobic membrane. Both hydrophilic and hydrophobic molecules can be found in liposomes because hydrophobic compounds are easily absorbed by lipid membranes. How far a medicine is positioned will depend on its lipid content and other physiochemical properties. When lipid bilayers combine with other cell bilayers (the cell membrane), liposomal contents are released, which subsequently deliver the required medication molecules to the site of action. The following factors contribute to the production of bilayers:

- Unfavourable interactions between the hydrophilic and hydrophobic phases can be mitigated by folding into closed, concentric vesicles.

- The massive free energy difference between the hydrophilic and hydrophobic environments is lessened by the formation of huge vesicles, due to the fact that spherical shapes have the least surface tension and are the most stable. The self-assembled structure that results in vesicles is therefore as stable as feasible.

Procedure for administering medication with liposomes:

1. *Adsorption*: The process of adsorption is how liposomes attach to cell membranes.

2. *Endocytosis*: The internalisation and engulfment of liposomes within the liposomes after their adsorption on the cell membrane.

3. *Fusion*: When liposomal lipid bilayers unite with the lipoidal cell membrane by lateral diffusion and lipid intermingling, liposome contents are directly delivered to the cytoplasm.

4. *Lipid exchange*: Because the phospholipids in the cell membrane and the liposomal lipid membrane are similar, lipid transfer proteins in the cell membrane can recognise liposomes and initiate lipid exchange.

For example, cancer cells need to consume enormous amounts of fat in order to meet their requirements for rapid development. They also recognise liposomes, which are filled with anticancer drugs, as a potential source of sustenance. When liposomes target them, they are absorbed. Anticancer medications destroy cancer cells as soon as they break free from the liposome and enter the location [16].

4. Classification of liposomes

Liposomes are categorised depending on the size and the number of bilayers. Unilamellar vesicles come in three different varieties: large (LUV), small (SUV), and multilamellar (MLV). Conventional liposomes (CL), pH-sensitive liposomes, cationic liposomes, long circulating liposomes (LCL), and immuno-liposomes are the different types of liposomes based on their composition. As illustrated in **Figure 2**, they are categorised as reverse phase evaporation vesicles (REV), French press vesicles (FPV), and ether injection vesicles (EIV) in accordance with the technique of preparation [17].

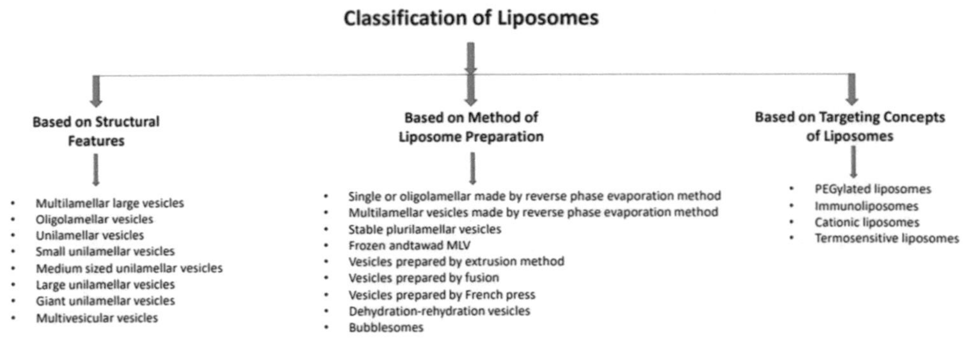

Figure 2.
Liposome classification.

5. Liposome stability

The stability of the liposomes throughout production, storage, and distribution determines the therapeutic efficacy of the drug molecule. The maintenance of the physical and chemical stability of the active molecule throughout the development and storage phases is ensured by a stable dosage form. In design-based stability tests, physical, chemical, and microbiological parameters are assessed, and product integrity is guaranteed throughout storage [18].

5.1 Physical stability

The size of the vesicles generated throughout the liposomal manufacturing stages varies. Vesicles assemble and enlarge to reach a thermodynamically favourable state during storage. Drug leakage from the vesicles during storage may cause fusion and breaking. The liposomal medicinal product's physical stability is lowered as a result. Therefore, vesicle size distribution and shape play a critical role in determining physical stability [19]. A variety of methods, including light scattering and electron microscopy, are employed to assess the morphology and size of the vesicles as well as their visual appearance. Although its content in the liposome structure cannot go above 50%, cholesterol reinforces the lipid membrane. Maintaining and stabilising the bioactive molecule at the liposome's centre is crucial. Maintaining pH levels and preventing excessive unsaturation of phospholipids during simple peroxidation are two ways to preserve physical stability. It is necessary to keep them chilled at 4°C to prevent freezing and exposure to light.

5.2 Chemical stability

Chemically unsaturated fatty acids known as phospholipids are prone to oxidation and hydrolysis, which could compromise the stability of the medicinal product. The stability of a liposomal formulation is greatly influenced by pH, ionic strength, solvent system, and buffering species. The production of hydroxy and cyclic peroxidases as a result of free radical generation during the oxidation process is known as oxidation degradation. To avert oxidative disintegration, liposomes can be shielded from sunlight, supplemented with antioxidants like butylated hydroxyl toluene (BHT) or α-tocopherol, manufactured in an inert atmosphere like nitrogen or argon, or treated with EDTA to remove traces of heavy metals [20]. Lyso-phosphatidylcholine is produced when the ester bond at the C-4 position of the glycerol moiety of phospholipids is hydrolysed. The liposomal contents' permeability is increased as a result. Therefore, it is essential to regulate the lysoPC limit in lysosomal pharmaceutical products. Phosphatidylcholine and lysoPC-free liposomes can be combined to achieve it [21].

6. Properties of liposomes

Liposomes are spherical vesicles consisting of one or more phospholipid bilayers, used in drug delivery and other applications due to their unique properties. Below are the key properties of liposomes:

6.1 Biocompatibility and biodegradability

Liposomes are biocompatible and biodegradable because they are made of phospholipids, which are also found in biological membranes. Their suitability for medication administration is improved and the danger of toxicity is reduced because of this feature [3].

6.2 Amphiphilicity

Both hydrophilic and hydrophobic areas are present in liposomes. Medications soluble in water can be encapsulated by the hydrophilic core, while medications soluble in lipids can be included by the hydrophobic bilayer. A large variety of medications can be delivered because of this dual capability [2].

6.3 Size and charge variability

Depending on the makeup of the phospholipids, liposomes can have a size ranging from 50 nm to several micrometres with a surface charge that is neutral, positively charged (cationic), or negatively charged (anionic). Their size and charge affect how quickly they circulate through the bloodstream and are absorbed by cells [22].

6.4 Controlled release of encapsulated drugs

Drugs that have been encapsulated can be released gradually and under control using liposomes. The liposomal membrane's composition can be altered to control this release, as can the use of stimuli-responsive components that release the medication in response to changes in temperature or pH [23].

6.5 Low immunogenicity

When liposomes are properly formed, such as by adding polyethylene glycol (PEGylation), they can elude the immune system and avoid being quickly cleared by the mononuclear phagocyte system (MPS). As a result, the drug's bioavailability is improved and its bloodstream circulation time is prolonged [24].

6.6 Encapsulation efficiency

Liposomes are highly effective at encapsulating pharmaceuticals that are hydrophilic, hydrophobic, or amphiphilic. They can thereby deliver a variety of therapeutic agents with greater versatility, enhancing medication solubility and stability, and lowering toxicity [25].

6.7 Enhanced permeability and retention (EPR) effect

Liposomes' increased permeability and retention effect allows them to accumulate in tumour tissues. Because the vascularisation of tumours is often more permeable than that of healthy tissues, liposomes can effectively and passively target tumour locations and deliver anticancer medications [26].

7. Advantages of liposomes

- *Biocompatibility and biodegradability:* Because liposomes are formed from natural phospholipids, the carriers themselves are biocompatible and biodegradable, with essentially no risk of toxicity, and they are easily metabolised within the body without causing harm to the host (**Figure 3**) [27].

- *Improved drug delivery:* Liposomes have the capacity to encapsulate both hydrophilic and hydrophobic pharmaceuticals, increase the solubility profiles of poorly soluble medications, and protect drugs from degradation. This increases the bioavailability and therapeutic index of the medicines [2].

- *Targeted delivery:* Liposomes can be modified to have surface ligands that allow them to target specific cells or tissues, reducing off-target effects while increasing drug accumulation at the intended region. This is especially advantageous in cancer therapy since targeting tumour cells can reduce systemic toxicity [28].

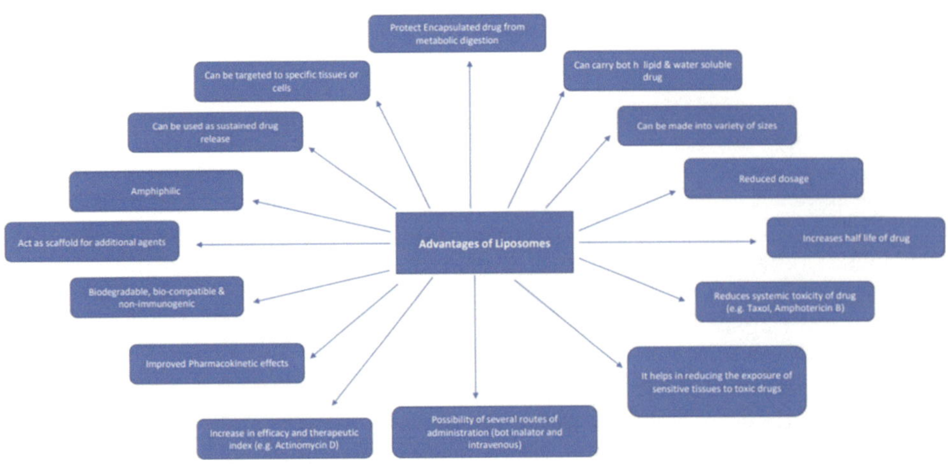

Figure 3.
Advantages of liposome [16].

- *Reduced toxicity:* This reduces the exposure of normal tissues to harmful medicines, lowering side effects and boosting patient tolerance [2].
- *Controlled release:* Liposomes can be engineered to release their components at a regulated and predetermined time, allowing medications to be delivered in a sustained form for a longer period of time, resulting in reduced frequency dosing and higher patient compliance [3].

8. Disadvantages of liposomes

- *Stability issues:* Liposomes are therefore susceptible to instability in terms of encapsulated drug leakage, fusion, and phospholipid oxidation, all of which significantly impair their effectiveness and shelf life [2].
- *High production costs:* Liposome synthesis and purification can be complex and expensive, which may limit their widespread application, particularly in resource-limited situations [29].
- *Rapid clearance by the reticuloendothelial system (RES):* Liposomes are quickly recognised and eliminated by the mononuclear phagocyte system (MPS) in the liver and spleen, potentially limiting their circulation time and efficacy [28].
- *Limited drug loading capacity:* The amount of pharmaceuticals that can be incorporated into liposomes may be limited depending on the type of liposome and the drug's qualities. This may have an impact on the dosages that can be administered [29].
- *Immunogenicity potential:* Liposomes, particularly non-PEGylated or unmodified ones, have the potential to stimulate the immune system, resulting in hypersensitivity reactions or accelerated clearance from the circulation [2].

9. Methods for preparation

The Bangham technique (thin film hydrolysis), ether/ethanol injection, reverse phase evaporation, detergent depletion, heating, microfluidic channel, membrane extrusion, homogenisation, and sonication are examples of conventional liposome synthesis techniques. Researchers have been using dual asymmetric freezing and freeze drying for almost 10 years. Supercritical fluid (SCF) and centrifugation (DAC) for the delivery of liposomal drugs. Drug delivery techniques that are cutting edge include lysolipid and depo-foam liposomes.

9.1 The Bangham method of thin film hydration

The Bangham technique was the first widely utilised technique to create liposomes [30, 31]. With this technique, lipids are dissolved in an organic solvent (dichloromethane, ethanol, chloroform, or a mixture of methanol and chloroform). The solvent that is organic is melted in a vacuum at 45–60°C to form a thin coating of lipid. After 2 hours of steady agitation in aqueous solutions at 60–70°C, the thin lipid layer swells and forms round, closed liposomes [32].

9.2 Methods of injecting ethanol/ether

In 1973, Batzri and Korn presented the ethanol injection technique [33]. Lipids are dissolved in an organic solvent (such as ethanol, diethyl ether, or an ether-methanol mixture) and then injected into an aqueous phase to create liposomes. At 55–65°C or with less pressure, encapsulate the material. Moreover, heating is necessary to extract the organic solvent from the liposomes since ether is incompatible with aqueous media [34]. The inkjet method was created by Hauschild et al. as a contemporary ethanol injection technique. Using this method, a drug solution, whether hydrophilic, lipophilic, or both, was dissolved in ethanol and converted into an inkjet device that allowed for the large-scale production of liposomes with remarkable control over particle size [35].

9.3 Method of reverse phase evaporation

The reverse phase evaporation method [36], developed by Szoka and Papahadjopoulos, involves dissolving medications in aqueous media and lipids in an organic solvent. After that, the mixture is sonicated to create inverted or emulsion-free micelles. A rotary evaporator is used to progressively evaporate the organic solvent, turning the micelles into a viscous or gel-like substance. The gel collapses at a crucial stage, releasing some inverted micelles. Liposomes are produced when more phospholipids surround the remaining micelles in a bilayer. A modified reverse-phase evaporation approach was proposed by Handa et al. [37], with the primary benefit being the liposome's excellent encapsulation.

9.4 Freeze-drying method

Liu et al. discovered the lyophilisation monophasic solution method for liposome manufacturing. This method involves dissolving the lipid and medicine in tert-butyl alcohol at 450°C, while the lyoprotectant dissolves in water. The two resulting solutions are combined to form a third identical monophasic solution, which is then filtered and freeze dried to produce proliposomes. The freeze-drying process consists of two steps. The substance is frozen at −40°C and dried at ambient temperature, yielding liposomes with a mean diameter of 100–300 nm [38].

9.5 Dual asymmetric centrifugation method (DAC)

In contrast to the standard centrifugation procedure, which calls for the vials to be rotated on their own centre axis, the DAC method involves rotating sealed vials on the main rotational axis at a defined speed and distance in addition to rotating on their own axis. The primary rotation forces the sample outward, and the adhesion between the sample and the rotating vial causes the revolution around its own centre to force the sample material in the opposite direction. Hence, mechanical turbulence and capitations introduce energy into the sample preparation process, resulting in the production of nano-liposomes with an optimum size distribution of approximately 60 nm [39].

9.6 Supercritical fluid methods (SCF)

Supercritical fluid extraction, supercritical-assisted liposome formation (super Lip) [40], depressurisation of an expanded liquid organic solution-suspension method (DELOS), supercritical anti-solvent method (SAS), supercritical reverse phase evaporation method (SCRPE), and particles from gases [41, 42] are examples of SCF methods that have been developed as green techniques to overcome the limitations of toxicity and degradability of conventional methods. Because it is inflammable, affordable, non-corrosive, non-toxic, acceptable to the environment, and appropriate for thermolabile chemicals, CO2 is the most often used supercritical gas [43].

9.7 Formation of liposomes

The following factors determine whether the liposome preparation technique is best:

- The physicochemical properties of the liposomal components and the substance to be entrapped;
- The imprisoned substance's effective concentration and possible toxicity;
- Extra procedures needed for the vesicles' application or delivery;
- The vesicles' ideal dimensions, polydispersity, and shelf life for the planned use; and,
- The ability to produce safe and effective liposomal products on a wide scale and the reproducibility of batch-to-batch production.

10. Characterisation of liposomes

10.1 Size and size distribution

When it comes to regulating the in vivo release of drug-loaded liposomes, vesicle size is crucial. Liposomes' average size is determined by their manner of production and phospholipid content.

Numerous methods are used to analyse size and size distribution, such as:

1. Microscopic methods include SEM, freeze-fracture TEM, negative stain TEM, and optical microscopy. Liposomes are imaged using SEM and TEM techniques, which are also utilised to measure the inter-bilayer distance and bilayer thickness [44]. Atomic force microscopy (AFM), a very high-resolution scanning probe microscopy that creates 3D micrographs with resolution of nanometres and A0 scale to analyse the liposome shape, stability, size, and dynamic process of lipid nano-capsules, is one of the recently developed microscopic techniques [45].

2. Hydrodynamic methods include gel exclusion chromatography, analytical centrifugation, field flow fractionation, ultracentrifugation, and others that are

used to analyse size distribution, elution properties, and liposome homogeneity in addition to estimating a compound's molecular mass [46].

3. Lipid vesicle size can be determined using diffraction light scattering techniques such quasi-elastic light scattering, laser light scattering, and photon correlation spectroscopy.

Liposomes smaller than 1 μm in size can have their mean diameter measured using these methods. Depending on whether a liposome formulation is intended for parenteral, topical, or inhalation application, it is important to keep an eye on its size. Liposomal size can be modified by a number of techniques, including homogenisation, extrusion, and sonication.

10.2 Calculating lamellarity

The quantity of lipid bilayers enclosing the lipid vesicles is known as lamellarity. Liposome size, homogeneity, and lamellarity can all be determined by means of cryo-electron microscopy, 31P-nuclear magnetic resonance (NMR), and small-angle X-ray scattering (SAXS) techniques [47].

10.3 Zeta potential

The main factor influencing cellular absorption and customised drug delivery is the zeta potential. By generating an electric field in response to incident laser scattering on moving particles, the laser Doppler electrophoresis and Zetasizer assess the zeta potential of liposomal dispersion. The zeta potential is affected by a number of variables, including pH, ionic strength, and particle concentration. The total surface charge and blood circulation time of liposomes are influenced by their lipid composition, specifically the positive- and negative-charged phospholipids [48].

10.4 Efficient encapsulation/entrapment

The percentage of water-soluble medicine and aqueous phase that are encapsulated during liposome production is known as encapsulation efficiency. The percentage of entrapment per milli gramme of lipid is how it should be shown. Drug bioavailability will increase with improved entrapment efficiency [49]. Solid phase extraction, size exclusion chromatography, hollow fibre centrifugal ultrafiltration and centrifugation ultrafiltration, mini-column centrifugation, and protamine aggregation are some of the techniques used to determine entrapment efficiency. Liposomes can be purified and separated using the mini-column centrifugation method; for negatively charged and neutral liposomes, the protamine aggregation method is employed. An indirect method of gauging encapsulation efficiency is to calculate the percentage of the drug's value that remains unencapsulated after being subtracted from the total amount to be used [50].

10.5 In vitro drug release studies

An in vitro diffusion cell or a dialysis bag is used for the 370°C in vitro drug release experiments. To replicate in vivo conditions, the cell or bag needs to be dampened with receptor media that contains pH 7.4 buffer and continuously agitated under sink conditions. A fresh medium volume was added to the receptor media at regular intervals, and the required amount of the medium was taken. The concentration was then assessed using UV-visible spectrophotometry and HPLC. The release of water-soluble drugs is influenced by the cholesterol concentration in liposomal formulations; an increase in cholesterol concentration accelerates the release of the drug [51].

10.6 In vivo performance

The pharmacokinetic characteristics of individual vesicles can impact the in vivo performance of liposome-containing drugs. Intravenous liposome delivery is used to examine the in vivo effectiveness of liposomal drug delivery methods by showing rapid clearance from the liver and spleen. Greater than 0.5 μm liposomes were phagocytosed, but liver parenchymal cells absorbed liposomes smaller than 0.1 μm. Liposomes with cholesterol increase stability by stopping drug leakage. Hyaluronic acid was used to functionalise magnetic liposome nanocomposites loaded with the anticancer medication imatinib. Fluorescence photos were obtained at 2, 4, and 8 hours after injecting these magnetic liposomes into a mouse model to examine their in vivo behaviour. When the fluorescence signal is at its highest, magnetic liposomes are absorbed and retained [52].

11. Applications of liposomes

Drug delivery systems: Liposomes are extensively employed as drug delivery vehicles for a wide range of drugs including anticancer agents, antibiotics, antifungal, and antiviral drugs. Drugs formulated in the form of liposomes are administered with the aim of enhancing their stability, solubility, and bioavailability, and reducing toxicity and side effects.

- *Anticancer therapy*: The wide use of liposomes is their application in the delivery of chemotherapy drugs such as doxorubicin (e.g., Doxil) and daunorubicin (e.g., DaunoXome). In this application, the drug is intended to be delivered to the target tumour cells, thus minimising systemic exposure to the drug and therefore reducing the side effects [53].

- *Antibiotic delivery*: Liposomal formulations have been shown to improve antibiotic delivery for drugs such as amphotericin B (AmBisome) in fungal infections. The liposomal form reduces the nephrotoxicity and some other adverse reactions to the drug [54].

Gene delivery: Liposomes can be used for delivering genetic materials, such as DNA, RNA, and small interfering RNA (siRNA), into cells for their use in gene therapy. This helps shield the genetic materials from degradation; enhance cellular uptake of the said material; and hence facilitate handling genetic disorders, cancers, and viral infections.

- *Gene therapy*: Liposomal gene delivery, which is also known as lipoplex, is currently used for the delivery of genes that either serve to replace a defective gene or suppress the expression of a harmful gene. Liposomes are under clinical trials to treat cystic fibrosis, haemophilia, and several cancers (**Table 1**) [55].

Disease	**Liposomal drug**	**Clinical applications**	**Outcome**	**References**
Systemic Fungal Infections	*AmBisome* (Liposomal Amphotericin B)	Treatment of cryptococcosis and candidiasis	Decreased nephrotoxicity and improved antifungal efficacy	[56]
Kaposi's Sarcoma	*Doxil* (Liposomal Doxorubicin)	Treatment of AIDS-related Kaposi's sarcoma	Improved tumour targeting and reduced systemic toxicity	[53]
Rheumatoid Arthritis	Liposomal Prednisolone	Anti-inflammatory therapy	Reduced inflammation with fewer side effects	[2]
Alzheimer's Disease	Liposomal Curcumin	Cognitive enhancement in Alzheimer's patients	Better brain penetration and reduced amyloid plaques	[57]
Breast Cancer	*Mylotarg* (Liposomal Gemtuzumab Ozogamicin)	Treatment of HER2-positive breast cancer	Enhanced targeting of cancer cells, leading to better outcomes	[58]
Hepatitis A	Liposomal Hepatitis A Vaccine	Preventive vaccine for hepatitis A infection	Enhanced immune response and prolonged protection	[59]
Cardiovascular Disease	Liposomal Statins	Targeted delivery for atherosclerosis management	Reduced plaque size and inflammation with fewer side effects	[60]
Pancreatic Cancer	Liposomal Irinotecan (*Onivyde*)	Treatment of metastatic pancreatic cancer	Improved overall survival and progression-free survival compared to standard therapy	[61]
Triple-Negative Breast Cancer	Liposomal Doxorubicin and Cyclophosphamide	Treatment of early-stage triple-negative breast cancer	Higher pathological complete response and better tolerability than free drugs	[62]
Non-Small Cell Lung Cancer (NSCLC)	Liposomal Cisplatin	Treatment of advanced NSCLC	Reduced nephrotoxicity and enhanced efficacy compared to free cisplatin	[63]
Ovarian Cancer	*Doxil* (Liposomal Doxorubicin)	Treatment of advanced ovarian cancer	Reduced cardiotoxicity and prolonged drug circulation	[64]
	Liposomal Paclitaxel	First-line treatment for ovarian cancer	Increased tumour response rate and reduced peripheral neuropathy compared to free paclitaxel	[65]
Colorectal Cancer	Liposomal Irinotecan (*Onivyde*) plus Fluorouracil and Leucovorin	Second-line treatment for metastatic colorectal cancer	Significantly improved survival compared to other irinotecan formulations	[66]

Disease	Liposomal drug	Clinical applications	Outcome	References
Glioblastoma	Liposomal Temozolomide	Treatment of recurrent glioblastoma	Enhanced brain tumour penetration and improved survival rates in clinical trials	[67]
HIV/AIDS (Kaposi's Sarcoma)	*Doxil* (Liposomal Doxorubicin)	Treatment of Kaposi's sarcoma in HIV patients	Reduced systemic toxicity and prolonged drug exposure	[68]
Prostate Cancer	Liposomal Docetaxel	Treatment of castration-resistant prostate cancer	Increased median survival and improved quality of life	[69]
Hepatocellular Carcinoma	Liposomal Doxorubicin	Advanced hepatocellular carcinoma treatment	Higher drug concentration in tumours with fewer side effects	[70]

Table 1.
Recent clinical examples of liposomal drug delivery systems.

Vaccine delivery: The usage of liposomes as adjuvants in vaccine formulations increases the immune response to antigens and allows for better vaccination. Liposomal vaccines can deliver antigens more efficiently and give sustained release, leading to prolonged immune stimulation.

- *COVID-19 vaccines*: The mRNA vaccines have used lipid nanoparticles to protect them from any form of degradation; these have included Pfizer-BioNTech and Moderna vaccines. These nanoparticles protect the mRNA from any form of degradation and at the same time facilitate its delivery into cells so that it may be used for generating the antigen that then provokes an immune response [71].

Cosmetics and dermatological applications: Liposomes are also used in cosmetic formulations to improve the delivery of active substances into the skin. They have been found to increase the stability and penetrability of vitamins, antioxidants, and moisturisers, hence presenting more effective cosmetics.

- *Anti-ageing creams*: The liposomes in the creams can act as carriers for the deeper penetration of retinoids, peptides, and other active molecules, thereby increasing their activity to diminish wrinkles and fine lines [72].

Diagnostic imaging: Liposomes can be filled with contrast agents and applied to various diagnostic imaging methods including MRI and nuclear imaging. Such liposomal contrast agent increases the visibility of tumours, inflamed tissues, or other pathological sites.

- *MRI contrast agents*: Gadolinium- or iron oxide nanoparticle-based liposomes are applied as contrast agents in MRI for improved imaging of tumours and other abnormalities in soft tissues [73].

Pulmonary delivery: Inhalable liposomal carriers allow for the targeting of drug delivery to the lungs and exhibit potential in treating specific respiratory diseases, such as asthma, chronic obstructive pulmonary disease (COPD), and lung infections.

- *Inhalation therapies*: Liposomes have been developed that encapsulate corticosteroids, antibiotics, and bronchodilators and deliver them precisely to the lungs. Such developed formulations might be beneficial in reducing the systemic side effects because of an increased local drug concentration [74].

12. Conclusion

Drug delivery systems are majorly advanced by liposomes, as they assure improved bioavailability of the therapeutic agents, their selective delivery, and reduced toxicity. In addition to encapsulating hydrophilic drugs, their ability to encapsulate hydrophobic drugs as well, coupled with excellent biocompatibility, makes them versatile carriers for a wide range of pharmaceutical applications. Although key challenges still remain on issues like stability, scalability, and cost-effectiveness, their potential continues to be enhanced with ongoing research and technological innovations in the field of liposomal therapies. As these continue to develop, liposomes have the potential to be a game-changing influence in the way that personalised medicine and treatment outcomes for many diverse medical specialties are approached.

Author details

Vaibhavi Patel* and Pranav Y. Dave
School of Engineering & Technology, National Forensic Sciences University, Gujarat, India

*Address all correspondence to: vaibhavipatel940@gmail.com

References

[1] Gregoriadis G. The carrier potential of liposomes in biology and medicine. New England Journal of Medicine. 1976;**295**(14):765-770

[2] Allen TM, Cullis PR. Liposomal drug delivery systems: From concept to clinical applications. Advanced Drug Delivery Reviews. 2013;**65**(1):36-48

[3] Torchilin VP. Recent advances with liposomes as pharmaceutical carriers. Nature Reviews Drug Discovery. 2005;**4**(2):145-160

[4] Immordino ML, Dosio F, Cattel L. Stealth liposomes: Review of the basic science, rationale, and clinical applications, existing and potential. International Journal of Nanomedicine. 2006;**1**(3):297

[5] Marchianoa V, Matosb M, Pertierraa ES, Gutiérrezb G, Blanco-Lópeza MC. Vesicles as antibiotic carrier: State of art. International Journal of Pharmaceutics. 2020;**585**:119478

[6] Cha Y, Son B, Ryu S. Efective removal of staphylococcal bioflms on various food contact surfaces by Staphylococcus aureus phage endolysin LysCSA13. Food Microbiology. 2019;**84**:103245

[7] Chunyan L, Zhang L, Zhu W, Guo R, Sun H, Chen X, et al. Barriers and stratagies of cationic liposomes for cancer gene therapy. Molecular Therapy-Methods and Clinical Development. 2020;**18**:751-764

[8] Rodrigues BS, Kanekiyo T, Singh J. In vitro and in vivo characterization of CPP and transferrin modifed liposomes encapsulating pDNA. Nanomedicine: Nanotechnology, Biology and Medicine. 2020;**28**:102225

[9] Bezerra CF, Alencar Junior JG, Honorato RL, Santos ATL. Antifungal activity of furnesol incorporated in liposomes and associated with fuconazole. Chemistry and Physics of Lipids. 2020;**233**:104987

[10] Oliveira JK, Nakamura TU, Correa AG, Petrilli R, Vianna Lopez RF, Nakamura CV, et al. Liposome-based nanocarrier loaded with a new quinoxaline derivative for the treatment of cutaneous leishmaniasis. Materials Science and Engineeting: C. 2020;**110**:110720

[11] Zhang Y, Wei H, Du Y, Ying D, Zhao C, Zhang Y, et al. Dimeric artesunate phospholipid-conjugated liposomes as promising anti-infammatory therapy for rheumatoid arthritis. International Journal of Pharmaceutics. 2020;**576**:119178

[12] Zhang ZJ, Michniak-Kohn B. Flavosomes, novel deformable liposomes for the co-delivery of anti-infammatory compounds to skin. International Journal of Pharmaceutics. 2020;**585**:119500

[13] Bai L, Fei WD, Ying YG, Miao H, Du F, Zhang WY, et al. Liposomes encapsulated iridium (III) polypyridyl complexes enhance anticancer activity in vitro and in vivo. Journal of Inorganic Biochemistry. 2020;**205**:111014

[14] Li Y, Tan X, Liu X, Liu L, Fang Y, Rao R, et al. Enhanced anticancer efect of doxorubicin by TPGS-coated liposomes with Bcl-2 siRNA-corona for dual suppression of drug resistance. Asian Journal of Pharmaceutical Sciences. 2020;**15**(5):646-660

[15] Kumar KS, Bhowmik D, Deb L. Recent trends in liposomes used As

novel drug delivery system. The Pharma Innovation. 2012;**1**(1, Part A):29

[16] Guimarães D, Cavaco-Paulo A, Nogueira E. Design of liposomes as drug delivery system for therapeutic applications. International Journal of Pharmaceutics. 2021;**601**:120571

[17] Akbarzadeh A, Rezaei-Sadabady R, Davaran S, Joo SW, Zarghami N, et al. Liposome: Classification, preparation and applications. Nanoscale Research Letters. 2013;**8**:102

[18] Yadav AV, Murthy MS, Shete AS, Sakhare S. Stability aspects of liposomes. Indian Journal Of Pharmaceutical Education And Research. 2011;**45**:402-413

[19] Grit M, Crommelin DJ. Chemical stability of liposomes: Implications for their physical stability. Chemistry and Physics of Lipids. 1993;**64**:3-18

[20] Çagdas M, Sezer AD, Bucak S. Liposomes as potential drug carrier systems for drug delivery. Nanotechnology and Nanomaterials. 2014;**2014**:1-50

[21] Cruz-Leal Y, Machado Y, López-Requena A, Canet L, Laborde R, et al. Role of B-1 cells in the immune response against an antigen encapsulated into phosphatidyl choline-containing liposomes. International Immunology. 2014;**26**:427-437

[22] Bozzuto G, Molinari A. Liposomes as nanomedical devices. International Journal of Nanomedicine. 2015;**10**:975-999

[23] Mura S, Nicolas J, Couvreur P. Stimuli-responsive nanocarriers for drug delivery. Nature Materials. 2013;**12**(11):991-1003

[24] Immordino ML, Dosio F, Cattel L. Stealth liposomes: Review of the basic science, rationale, and clinical applications. International Journal of Nanomedicine. 2006;**1**(3):297-315

[25] Pattni BS, Chupin VV, Torchilin VP. New developments in liposomal drug delivery. Chemical Reviews. 2015;**115**(19):10938-10966

[26] Maeda H, Wu J, Sawa T, Matsumura Y, Hori K. Tumor vascular permeability and the EPR effect in macromolecular therapeutics: A review. Journal of Controlled Release. 2000;**65**(1-2):271-284

[27] Patil YP, Jadhav S. Liposomes: Fundamentals, properties, and applications in drug delivery. Cell Biochemistry and Biophysics. 2021;**44**(2):153-167

[28] Sercombe L, Veerati T, Moheimani F, Wu SY, Sood AK, Hua S. Advances and challenges of liposome assisted drug delivery. Frontiers in Pharmacology. 2015;**6**:286

[29] Bulbake U, Doppalapudi S, Kommineni N, Khan W. Liposomal formulations in clinical use: An updated review. Pharmaceutics. 2017;**9**(2):12

[30] Bangham AD, Standish MM, Watkins JC. Diffusion of univalent ions across the lamellae of swollen phospholipids. Journal of Molecular Biology. 1965;**13**(1):238-252

[31] Bangham AD, Standish MM, Weissmann G. The action of steroids and streptolysin S on the permeability of phospholipid structures to cations. Journal of Molecular Biology. 1965;**13**(1):253-259

[32] Zhang H. Thin flm hydration followed by extrusion method for

liposome preparation. Methods in Molecular Biology. 2017;**1522**:17-22

[33] Batzri S, Korn ED. Single bilayer liposomes prepared without sonication. Biochimica et Biophysica Acta (BBA) – Biomembranes. 1973;**298**(4):1015-1019

[34] Deamer DW. Preparation and properties of ether injection liposomes. Annals of the New York Academy of Sciences. 1978;**308**:250-258

[35] Bnyan R, Cesarini L, Khan I, Roberts M, Ehtezazi T. The efect of ethanol evaporation on the properties of inkjet produced liposomes. DARU Journal of Pharmaceutical Sciences. 2020;**28**(5):275-298

[36] Szoka F, Papahadjopoulos D. Procedure for preparation of liposomes with large internal aqueous space and high capture by reverse-phase evaporation. Proceedings of the National Academy of Sciences of the USA. 1978;**75**(9):4194-4198

[37] Handa T, Naito S, Hiramatsu M, Tsuboi M. Thermal SiO and H13CO+ line observations of the dense molecular cloud G0.11-0.11 in the galactic center region. The Astrophysical Journal. 2006;**636**:261-266. 55

[38] Yen TTH, Dan LN, Hoang LD, Tung BT, Minh Hue PT. Preparation and characterization of freeze dried liposomes loaded with amphotericin B. Current Drug Therapy. 2019;**14**(1):12

[39] Hirsch M, Ziroli V, Helm M, Massing U. Preparation of small amounts of sterile siRNA – Liposomes with high entrapping efciency by dual asymmetric centrifugation (DAC). Journal of Controlled Release. 2009;**135**(1):80-88

[40] Maja L, Zeljko K, Mateja P. Sustainable technologies for liposome preparation. The Journal of Supercritical Fluids. 2020;**165**:1049-1084

[41] Trucillo P, Campardelli R, Scognamiglio M, Reverchon E. Control of liposomes diameter at micrometric and nanometric level using a supercritical assisted technique. Journal of CO2 Utilization. 2019;**32**:119-127. 7

[42] Chakravarty P, Famili A, Nagapudi K, Al-Sayah MA. Using supercritical fuid technology as a green alternative during the preparation of drug delivery systems. Pharmaceutics. 2019;**11**:629

[43] Primozic M, Colnik M, Knez Z, Leitgeb M. Advantages and disadvantages of using SC CO2 for enzyme release from halophilic fungi. Journal of Supercritical Fluids. 2019;**143**:286-293

[44] Lara LA, Avila EM, Gutierrez MAL, Alvarez EO, Olive KI. Radiolabeled liposomes and lipoproteins as lipidic nanoparticles for imaging and therapy. Chemistry and Physics of Lipids. 2020;**230**:104934

[45] Spyratou E, Mourelatou EA, Makropoulou M, Demetzos C. Atomic force microscopy: A tool to study the structure, dynamics and stability of liposomal drug delivery systems. Expert Opinion on Drug Delivery. 2009;**6**(3):305-317

[46] Mehdi Hasan M, Hasan M, Mondal JC, Hasan MA, Talukder S, Rashid HA. Liposomes: An advance tools for novel drug delivery system. The Pharma Innovation Journal. 2017;**6**(11):304-311

[47] Bokrova J, Marova I, Matouskova P, Pavelkova R. Fabrication of novel PHB-liposome nanoparticles and study on their toxicity in vitro.

Journal of Nanoparticle Research. 2019;**21**(3):256-289

[48] Smith MC, Crist RM, Clogston JD, McNeil SE. Zeta potential: A case study of cationic, anionic and neutral liposomes. Analytical and Bioanalytical Chemistry. 2017;**409**(24):5779-5787

[49] Ong SGM, Ming LC, Lee KS. Infuence of the encapsulation efciency and size of liposome on the oral bioavailability of griseofulvin-loaded liposomes. Pharmaceutics. 2016;**8**(3):25

[50] Moghimipour E, Handali S. Utilization of thin flm method for preparation of celecoxib loaded liposomes. Advanced Pharmaceutical Bulletin. 2012;**2**(1):93-98

[51] Shamshiri MK, Jaafari MR, Badiee A. Preparation of liposomes containing IFN-gamma and their potentials in cancer immunotherapy: In vitro and in vivo studies in a colon cancer mouse model. Life Sciences. 2021;**264**:11860-11865

[52] Amiri M, Gholami T, Amiri O, Pardakhti A, Ahmadi M, Akbari A, et al. The magnetic inorganic-organic nanocomposite based on ZnFe2O4 Imatinib-liposome for biomedical applications, in vivo and in vitro study. Journal of Alloys and Compounds. 2020;**849**:15660-15664

[53] Barenholz Y. Doxil®—The first FDA-approved nano-drug: Lessons learned. Journal of Controlled Release. 2012;**160**(2):117-134

[54] Wasan EK, Rosenblum MG, Yung A. Liposomal formulation of amphotericin B: Pharmacokinetic and efficacy evaluation. Journal of Antimicrobial Chemotherapy. 2009;**64**(4):771-780

[55] Nayerossadat N, Maedeh T, Ali PA. Viral and nonviral delivery systems for gene delivery. Advanced Biomedical Research. 2012;**1**:27

[56] Ellis JA. The immunology of the bovine respiratory disease complex. Veterinary Clinics of North America: Food Animal Practice. 2001;**17**(3):535-550

[57] Liu J, Wang F. Role of neuroinflammation in amyotrophic lateral sclerosis: Cellular mechanisms and therapeutic implications. Frontiers in Immunology. 2017;**8**:1005

[58] Godwin JL, Hoffman-Censits J, Plimack E. Recent developments in the treatment of advanced bladder cancer. In: Urologic Oncology: Seminars and Original Investigations. Vol. 36, No. 3. Elsevier; 2018. pp. 109-114

[59] Guo X, Zhong JY, Li JW. Hepatitis C virus infection and vaccine development. Journal of Clinical and Experimental Hepatology. 2018;**8**(2):195-204

[60] Zhao M, Woodward M, Vaartjes I, Millett ER, Klipstein-Grobusch K, Hyun K, et al. Sex differences in cardiovascular medication prescription in primary care: A systematic review and meta-analysis. Journal of the American Heart Association. 2020;**9**(11):e014742

[61] Wang-Gillam et al. Nanoliposomal Irinotecan with fluorouracil and folinic acid in metastatic pancreatic cancer after previous gemcitabine-based therapy. The Lancet. 2016;**387**(10018):545-557. DOI: 10.1016/S0140-6736(15)00986-1

[62] Mouridsen HT et al. Efficacy and safety of liposomal doxorubicin and cyclophosphamide in neoadjuvant chemotherapy for triple-negative breast cancer. Breast Cancer Research and Treatment. 2020;**180**(1):163-170. DOI: 10.1007/s10549-020-05530-7

[63] Li Y et al. Liposomal cisplatin versus standard cisplatin in patients with advanced non-small cell lung cancer. Journal of Thoracic Oncology. 2020;**15**(4):513-522. DOI: 10.1016/j.jtho.2019.12.010

[64] Gabizon AA. Liposome circulation time and tumor targeting: Implications for cancer chemotherapy. Advanced Drug Delivery Reviews. 1995;**16**(2-3):285-294

[65] Gradishar WJ et al. Phase III trial of liposomal paclitaxel compared to solvent-based paclitaxel for first-line treatment of ovarian cancer. Journal of Clinical Oncology. 2018;**36**(15):1574-1582. DOI: 10.1200/JCO.2017.75.5276

[66] Fuchs CS et al. Fluorouracil, leucovorin, and nanoliposomal irinotecan for metastatic colorectal cancer after prior therapy. New England Journal of Medicine. 2019;**379**(3):234-245. DOI: 10.1056/NEJMoa1812444

[67] Yang W et al. Liposomal temozolomide for recurrent glioblastoma: Improved drug delivery to brain tumors. Clinical Cancer Research. 2021;**27**(9):2515-2524. DOI: 10.1158/1078-0432.CCR-20-2475

[68] Stewart MA et al. Liposomal doxorubicin for Kaposi's sarcoma in HIV patients: A clinical perspective. AIDS Research and Human Retroviruses. 2021;**37**(4):324-330. DOI: 10.1089/AID.2020.0119

[69] De Bono JS et al. Liposomal docetaxel for castration-resistant prostate cancer: Results from a phase III trial. European Urology. 2022;**82**(2):180-188. DOI: 10.1016/j.eururo.2021.10.015

[70] Brown AJ et al. Liposomal doxorubicin for advanced hepatocellular carcinoma: A clinical trial analysis. Liver Cancer. 2023;**12**(2):289-299. DOI: 10.1159/000527495

[71] Hassett KJ, Benenato KE, Jacquinet E, Lee A, Woods A, Yuzhakov O, et al. Optimization of lipid nanoparticles for intramuscular administration of mRNA vaccines. Molecular Therapy-Nucleic Acids. 2019;**15**:1-11

[72] Morganti P, Fabrizi G, James B, Morganti G. Nanoliposome and other encapsulated nanoparticles: Cosmetic and therapeutic use. Journal of Applied Cosmetology. 2011;**29**(1):1-24

[73] Kou L, Sun J, Zhai Y, He Z. The endocytosis and intracellular fate of nanomedicines: Implication for rational design. Asian Journal of Pharmaceutical Sciences. 2017;**8**(1):1-10

[74] Kunda NK, Alfagih IM, Miyaji EN, Edwards AD. Liposomes as a carrier for pulmonary delivery of vaccines. Expert Opinion on Drug Delivery. 2015;**12**(11):1833-1847

Chapter 5

The Role of Percolation Theory: Can Formulations be Considered as *In-Organic Life* Administered to *Organic Life*?

Hans Leuenberger, Stephan Schmidt, Go Kimura, Michael Levin and Ofer Aqua

Abstract

The authors propose a new compelling concept and framework for understanding the human body as a dynamic, open thermodynamic system far from equilibrium conditions. This concept can be called "University of Florida College of Pharmacy Interpretation of Life-Sciences" by describing the human being as a model of a human supercomputer. The computer hardware only can function in a thermodynamic system with an influx of energy. Thus, the existence of life is directly related to a local reduction of the entropy leading to an "order out of chaos." Percolation theory allows predicting a system of "higher order" such as a pharmaceutical formulation leading to a specific disintegration time of tablets. The authors of this book chapter coined this ability as "In-organic Life", able to interact with "Organic Life". This concept leads to the conclusions: 1) The human body is not only sensitive to a single well defined drug, but also to combinations with n>= 2 safe generic drugs opening new research avenues for drug discovery and that the number of preclinical and animal studies can be reduced, 2) the human body is sensitive to a viral infection, and 3) to "friendly viral infections" attacking only antibiotic resistant bacteria or cancer cells as "phage" therapy. It is important to replace the current research concept of "reductionism" from complex to simple by an approach from "simple to complex". The storage of electromagnetic energy by using the Anderson localization will lead to a safe treatment of radioactive waste preventing it from being buried for thousands of years. Stauffer and Aharoni describe the Anderson localization as a super localization event. Thus, quantum percolation forms a bridge between the quantum mechanical approach describing (living and dead) matter as a collection of harmonic oscillators. It is important to realize that percolation theory defines coherence and coherence length.

Keywords: what is life?, digital twin, virtual patient, model-informed drug development (MIDD), University of Florida College of pharmacy interpretation of life-sciences, Anderson localization, reductionism

1. Introduction and state of the art

Pharmacometrics is the major task of the Center of Pharmacometrics and Systems Pharmacology (CPSP) and has evolved from a descriptive science to an applied science that has been increasingly used in all phases of drug development over the last decades. Today's application for accelerating and streamlining drug development is known as model-informed drug development (MIDD) or, model-informed drug discovery [1]. It is important to get acquainted with the following often used and cited abbreviations of foundational technical skills such as ADME (Absorption, Distribution, Metabolism, Excretion) principles, and NLME (Non-Linear Mixed Effects) modeling, PK (Pharmacokinetics), PD (Pharmacodynamics), and disease progression models. i.e. Mechanistic PK and PD models including PBPK (Physiologically Based Pharmacokinetic Modeling), a successful pharmacometrician should be an effective communicator, be able to think strategically, and be able to influence team-based decisions, as outlined in **Figure 1**.

This CPSP approach [1–4] has a lot of advantages being described to the public in the educational program of the University of Florida Winter School [4]. It is evident that the goal of CPSP is to strengthen the research activities for the benefit of the patients. The UF Winter School is an important platform for the exchange of views in optimizing the CPSP research activities.

In this context, it must be kept in mind that the existing scientific approach is governed by the concept of reductionism, "From Complex to Simple", with the disadvantage that this method may lead to a loss of information.

2. Development of a new scientific approach as a model for the human being: The impact of percolation theory and the order of a system

In the following section, we discuss the potential of the human being described as a supercomputer to be used as a model for a Virtual Patient. This approach is new but far from being mature. Additional effort to optimize this model is necessary. On the other hand, it must be mentioned that this innovative model simulates a "living biological system", since it represents an open physical system with influx of energy.

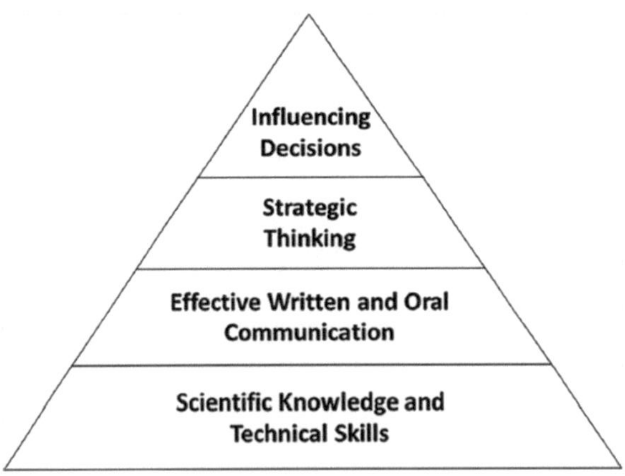

Figure 1.
Hierarchical skill set for pharmacometricians to successfully apply model-informed drug discovery and Development (MIDD) approaches [1].

According to the work [5, 6] of Nobel Laureate Ilya Prigogine such an open system with influx of energy allows the creation of life, respectively, the creation of a higher order. The latter reverses the classical "time arrow" which is defined by the second law of thermodynamics [5, 6] that the disorder (entropy) is constantly increasing. In other words, the model of the "human, organic supercomputer" [7] must include the following properties of a "supercomputer": (A) The hardware (the human body) being subject to aging, since the second law of thermodynamics cannot be switched off. (B) On the other hand, the cells in our body are replaced every 7 to 10 years. Interestingly, the definition of the "time arrow" based on the concept of entropy, leads to the conclusion that it is possible to define a system which can be coined as "inorganic life" [7] for a limited number of degrees of freedom to describe a "higher order".

Unfortunately, the "number of letters of the existing alphabet of inorganic chemistry is limited compared to organic chemistry using the DNA as letter and building blocks for the storage of information = code of life" [8].

However, the "replacement times" show a high variability of the different human organs of our body. Some human blood cells last only 2 days, while the cells in the middle of our eye lenses are not replaced at all during our life. Evidently, thanks to the open system with influx of energy, human cells, as a basic unit of a living organ, can be substituted. Lizards even can reconstruct lost tails. Interestingly, if the human liver is partly removed in a surgery, the missing liver cells can be replaced. This is an exception.

It is important to realize that the creation of a pharmaceutical formulation also can be considered as a "system of higher order". In this context, the highly disordered powder system consisting of particles of the active ingredient and functional excipients such as binder, disintegrant, filler, lubricant is designed as a drug delivery system such as a tablet showing a specific drug release. This property can be interpreted as a higher order of the tablet system.

It is important to note that the tablet properties can be modeled using percolation theory. Thus, percolation theory provides us with an equation by reversing the "time arrow" [6] of the second law of thermodynamics. Stauffer and Ahorni [9] included in their book "Introduction to Percolation Theory" a chapter on quantum percolation which triggers the hypothesis whether we have at the percolation threshold a superposition of two different quantum states? In principle, this could also happen at room temperature [7, 8]. Thus, the superposition of percolation thresholds at room temperature may allow us to use such a system as an analog quantum computer [8]. However, this hypothesis needs to be validated. In the optimal case, the human brain has the potential to perform such calculations.

In the case of a formulation, such an approach should lead to new insights for quality assurance purposes.

3. The potential of the new model to simulate the human being as supercomputer to be used as a virtual patient

As mentioned in the introduction, the basic equation of percolation theory can be used for the prediction of a quality assurance property of a higher-ordered system such as the tensile strength, deformation hardness or the elastic modulus of a tablet or its disintegration time. This feature is an intrinsic property of the basic equation of percolation theory such as Eq. (1) for the case of the tablet quality attribute "disintegration time". Due to the achieved higher order this result can be interpreted as a local reduction of the entropy *with the focus on local,* since the product also is subject to aging and to the second law of thermodynamics!

This local higher order can be coined to some extent by the author as "inorganic life" [7], since this process leads to a higher order as in the case of forming a highly ordered inorganic crystal.

Due to the lower number of degrees of freedom of inorganic chemistry compared to organic chemistry, the order in an inorganic crystal is limited regarding the content of information, which is defined by the crystal classes.

In other words, organic chemistry was able to create a comprehensive alphabet to store information based on DNA (**Figure 2**). This information can also be interpreted as an instruction, respectively as "software" [7], which represents the highest order of information!

Go Kimura used the basic equation of percolation theory to predict the hardness and the disintegration time of his tablets during his PhD thesis [10] at the University of Basel. In this context, he used as the critical exponent the value he obtained using non-linear regression analysis and *not a universal critical exponent, which is generally accepted.*

At the same time, Go Kimura used in his PhD thesis the Formulation Compute-Aided Design (F-CAD) by CINCAP [11]. He also successfully introduced F-CAD at his company Shionogi in Japan. For simplicity, we will use in the following equation of percolation theory to predict the tablet disintegration time as "order" parameter.

The application of the basic percolation equation to replace individual cells (= microprocessors) of an organ is a challenging next step, requiring additional concepts to complete the model of the human supercomputer as Virtual Patient.

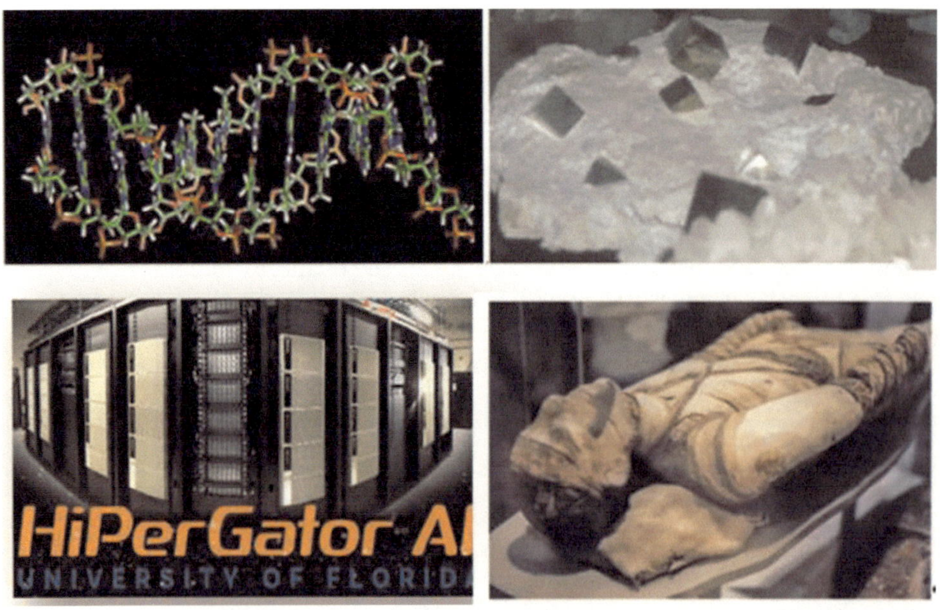

Figure 2.
The human supercomputer as Virtual Patient [7] with the Genetic DNA Code (top left) as software and the body (below right) as computer hardware simulating a supercomputer consisting of microprocessor (below left). Inorganic crystals are coined as "inorganic" life (top right).

The scientific community is invited to participate in this challenging journey. As mentioned in the introduction, the use of an open thermodynamic model with influx of energy locally allows the reduction of the entropy leading to a higher order of the system [7]. This is true in the field of inorganic and organic chemistry. In the case of inorganic chemistry this event was coined as "inorganic" life [7].

3.1 Disintegration time as a critical tablet quality attribute

A higher ordered system such as a tablet with a specific order parameter defining as an example the tablet disintegration time TD_{is} can be described by the basic equation of percolation theory [9]:

$$TD_{is} = SF\,(p - p_c)^{q^*} \text{ with } q^* = 2 \tag{1}$$

The variable p (= probability = relative density ρ_r) and p_c = percolation threshold, respectively critical relative density. Please note that q^* = 2 corresponds to the *universal critical exponent.* q^* = 2 is identical with the Einstein critical exponent for conductivity in 3D, SF = scaling factor.

Hans Leuenberger's former PhD student Rene Luginbuehl [12] did not have the opportunity to validate this conjecture, respectively hypothesis using a tablet formulation consisting of more than two ingredients. Eq. (1) describes the local reduction of entropy, increasing the degree of order and demonstrates a reversal of the "time arrow". In this context, Eq. (1) impresses by its simplicity.

Thus, the following fact needs to be kept in mind. The beauty of the deterministic classical Newtonian and the physics of Einstein is related to a minimum number of short and elegant equations to describe the natural phenomena such as force F = mass times acceleration, i.e. $F = m(d^2x/d^2t)$; kinetic energy E_k = function of mass and velocity, i.e. $E_k = 1/2(m\,[dx/dt]^2)$ and $E = mc^2$ that mass m is equivalent to an energy.

The contrary of a deterministic description is the end of certainty, the relativistic description of time, and that the mystery of the arrow of time is related to the constant increase of entropy in a closed thermodynamic system.

Thus, we need to get acquainted with the theory of chaos, bifurcation events and new laws in nature being difficult to describe with elegant short solutions! In the best case, we can write some more simple approximative equations describing the complex phenomenon or need to accept that the more elegant description is limited to a limited number of cases such as for "inorganic" life!

At the same time, we need to realize that the basic percolation equation is very flexible, using only four variables such as scaling factor, SF, probability p, percolation threshold p_c and the universal critical exponent q^*. If we introduce in this equation a dynamic percolation threshold, it may be possible to also describe events of organic life such as the continuous replacement of blood cells. Is our description using as virtual patient a "human supercomputer" as model sufficient?

Interestingly, Einstein was not convinced that the successful concept of quantum mechanics was complete. The creation of the concept of quantum mechanics started with the Copenhagen interpretation [13]. As an alternative, t' Hooft [14] proposed the cellular automaton interpretation of quantum mechanics, leading to additional questions such as whether an absolute vacuum can be found in the universe.

On the other hand, the successful mathematical language for the description of quantum mechanical systems leads to the question whether biological systems also

Tablet (Loading volume of MA, % v/v)	Disintegration time (sec.) (*n* = 3)
A (0)	550 ± 23
B (12.0)	596 ± 8
C (23.5)	616 ± 6
D (34.5)	604 ± 21
E (45.0)	428 ± 16
F (55.1)	266 ± 8
G (64.8)	453 ± 24
H (74.1)	758 ± 15

Table 1.
Disintegration time of mefenamic acid (MA) tablet formulations A-H according to the publication of Go Kimura [10].

need a different set of mathematical tools for a better understanding? (**Table 1**). The Standard Model and the Theory of Everything. The Standard Model is based on two pillars , that is, (1) Einstein's topic of General Relativity as a theoretical framework for understanding the universe in regions of both large scale and high mass such as planets, stars, galaxies including the gravitational forces of Newton and of classical physics, and (2) on the Quantum Mechanics as a theoretical framework that focuses on three non-gravitational forces in regions of both very small scale and low mass: subatomic particles, atoms and molecules covering the non-gravitational strong nuclear, weak nuclear and electromagnetic forces. According to Einstein, the framework of Quantum Mechanics is not complete. Thus, the Theory of Everything, an all-encompassing, coherent theoretical framework of physics that fully explains the universe is still missing. We cannot explain dark matter, the dark energy, etc. *Einstein was right, since the work of Dr Angelo Comunetti* [8] *showed that the electromagnetic forces are also valid in the subatomic region and should be correctly coined as third electromagnetic nuclear force since electromagnetic energy can be stored in a "localized" state of the nuclear wave function. In other words, it is important to note that the strength of this electromagnetic nuclear force is close to the nuclear strong force but should be distinguished from the "normal" electromagnetic interaction. For this reason, it is not possible to use neutron activation analysis to detect Au in such a "localized" state of the nuclear wave function*. Indeed, this electromagnetic nuclear force is initiating a Bose Einstein Condensate of photons at room temperature in bi-distilled water which can be considered as a semiconductor [8]. In addition, we must admit that we are primarily used studying our environment as a closed physical system without an influx of energy. Thus, the open physical system with influx of energy leads to different solutions. In the optimal case the Theory of Everything will include the concept "University of Florida College of Pharmacy Interpretation of Life-Sciences".

But let us first discuss the quality attribute "disintegration time" of a tablet in case of mefenamic acid (MA) tablets (**Figure 3**).

The values for r^2(= Pearson Correlation Coefficient) are 0.998 for **Figure 4a**, respectively, 0.996 for **Figure 4b**.

According to the above results, it can be expected that the non-linear regression analysis will lead to a percolation threshold close to ρ_c = 0.842 (**Table 2**). Thus, after linearization of Eq. (1), the following model can be applied as a rough approximation = linearization method for using a linear regression analysis:

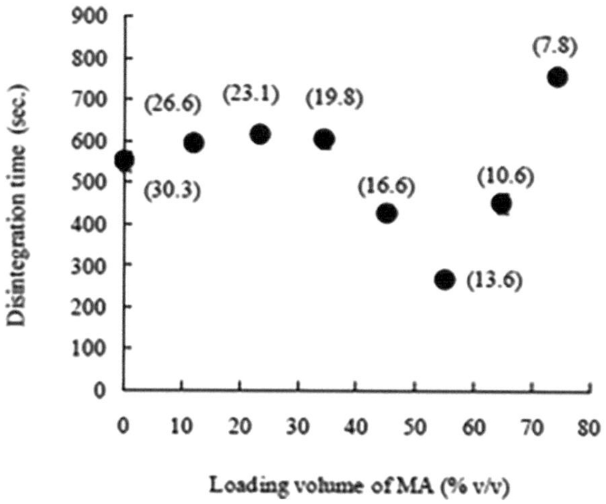

Figure 3.
Disintegration time of MA (mefenamic acid) tablet formulations A-H published by Dr. Go Kimura [10].

$$\mathrm{Sqr}(\mathrm{TD_{is}}) = 1222.8–1452.1\ \rho_r \qquad (2)$$

with ρ_r = relative density of the compact and ρ_r = 1-ε with ε = porosity, and with ρ_c = 1222.8/1452.1 = percolation threshold = 0.842.

$$\mathrm{TD_{is}} = (1222.8)^2\ (\rho_r - 0.842) \qquad (3)$$

However, this approximation does not correctly predict the $\mathrm{TD_{is}}$(R) results for ρ_c = 0.833 of **Table 3** for the tablets F, F′, G, G’ and H. For this reason, it makes sense to use for the model the percolation threshold ρ_c = 0.842 (after linearization based on **Table 4**), being close to the value of ρ_c = 0.841 of the non-linear regression analysis.

In addition, according to percolation theory, the shape of the quadratic function describing the minimum of the disintegration time should be symmetric. Thus, the following $\mathrm{TD_{is}}$ values for *lower relative densities* of tablets D*, D*’ E* and E*‘as mentioned in **Table 4** can be expected (**Figure 5**), assuming a slightly higher porosity after relaxation.

Please note that the rigorous application of percolation theory requests that Eq. (1) is symmetric with respect to the relative density ρ_r, leading to $\mathrm{TD_{is}}$ = 0 for ρ_r = 0.84144 = ρ_c.

However, **Figure 6a** and **b** shows an asymmetric behavior of the left and right-side branch of the $\mathrm{TD_{is}}$ results, leading to two different percolation threshold values ρ_c = 0.833, respectively ρ_c = 0.858.

This result does not make sense and may be due to the relaxation process of a system far from thermodynamic equilibrium in the spirits of Nobel Laureate Ilya Prigogine and to the lack of additional data regarding the relative densities and the use of interpolated values for the relative densities of **Tables 4** and 5.

In other words, it is important to study quantitatively relaxation processes for the validation of Eq. (1) with the universal critical exponent q^* = 2 for $\mathrm{TD_{is}}$.

Interestingly, the asymmetric behavior of the left and right-side branches of the quadratic Eq. (1) may also be responsible for the constant term 338 sec in the following equation:

$$\mathrm{TDis} = 7031096\ (\rho_{r,} - 0.84144)^2 + 338 \qquad (4)$$

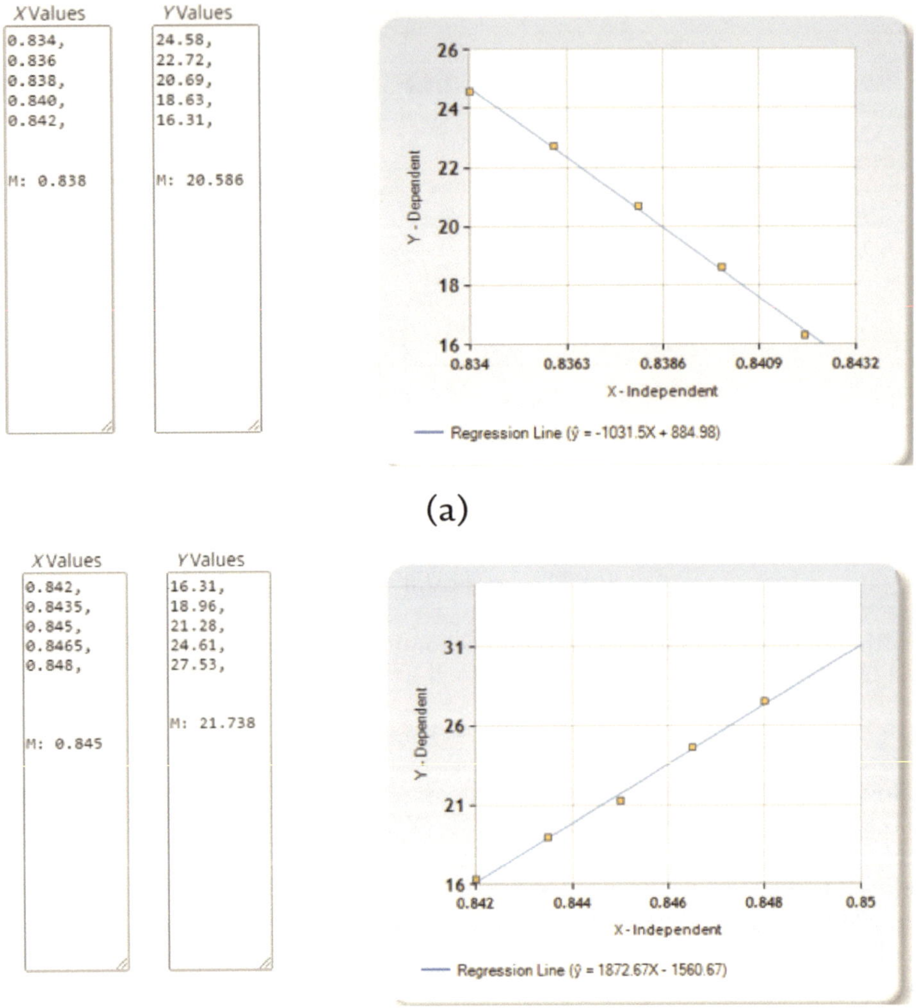

Figure 4.
*(a) Linear regression (left side L) based on the data from [12]. The values for r^2 (= Pearson correlation coefficient) are 0.998 for **Figure 4a**. (b) Linear regression (right side R) based on the data from [12]. The value for r^2 (= Pearson correlation coefficient) is equal to 0.996 for **Figure 4b**.*

of the non-linear regression analysis of **Figure 5**. In this context, the value ρ_c = 0.84144 is reasonable and was obtained by using the linear regression analysis.

Please note that Eq. (1) with the *universal* critical exponent q* [15] is *successfully* used *for the first time* for the quantitative description of the tablet quality attribute *disintegration time* TD_{is} for pharmaceutical formulations *consisting of more than two ingredients* [12].

According to the work of Prigogine the compression of disordered particles/granules is a thermodynamic process in an open system with influx of energy far from equilibrium conditions. Thus, it is important that the system has time to relax and that the quality attributes such as porosity of the final tablet, the tensile strength or the disintegration time are measured after ca 24 h, not earlier.

Tablet X Form	Rel. Dens. (L)	TD_{is} (L) (sec)	Sqr [TD_{is}(L)]	Tablet X Form	Rel Dens. (R)	TD_{is} (R) (sec)	Sqr [TD_{is}(R)]
D	0.834	604	24.58	F	0.842	266	16.31
D′	0.836	516	22.72	F′	0.8435	359.5	18.96
E	0.838	428	20.69	G	0.845	453	21.28
E'	0.840	347	18.63	G'	0.8465	605.5	24.61
F	0.842	266	16.31	H	0.848	758	27.53

*Eq. (1) was treated on both sides by taking the square root for using the linear regression analysis. The corresponding results are summarized in **Figure 6a** and **b**, leading to a percolation threshold ρ_c = 0.84144 = 884.98/1031.5 = 0.858 {left = side} respectively, ρ_c = 0.84144 = 1560.7/1872.7 = 0.833 (right-side).*

Table 2.
Data from [10], in blue = interpolated, in red = extrapolated value.

Tablet X Form	Rel. Dens. (L)	TD_{is} (L) (sec)	Predicted Result (sec)	Tablet X Form	Rel Dens. (R)	TD_{is} (R) (sec)	Predicted Result (sec)
D	0.834	604	451	F	0.842	266	284
D′	0.836	516	379	F′	0.8435	359.5	387
E	0.838	428	313	G	0.845	453	505
E'	0.840	347	254	G'	0.8465	605.5	639
F	0.842	266	284	H	0.848	758	789

Experimental and predicted results based on Eq. (1). Evidently, the predicted results based on the calculated percolation threshold ρ_c = 0.833 (left side) lead to better results than in case of ρ_c = 0.858 (right = side).

Table 3.
Data from [10], in blue = interpolated, in red = extrapolated value.

For this reason, it cannot be excluded that the porosity of the tablets, respectively, the relative densities of D, D′, E and E' were measured before the tablets were fully relaxed. However, this hypothesis had to be validated in future studies.

It is important to note that the basic percolation equation does not replace the successful software F-CAD (= Formulation – Computer-Aided Design) by CINCAP [11], which was introduced at the Pharmaceutical Company SHIONOGI by Go Kimura [10]. In his PhD thesis [10], he used F-CAD and was able to predict the disintegration time of MA tablets, as shown in **Table 6**.

3.2 The Young's elastic modulus as a critical tablet quality attribute

Another example of "inorganic" life can also be described by the basic percolation equation for the table quality attribute "elastic young modulus" f of the tablet, respectively, deformation hardness or tensile strength. In the case that no capping of tablets takes place, all three quality attributes show a proportionality [17]:

$$\text{Elastic Modulus f} = \text{SF}\ (\text{p–p}_\text{c})^{\text{q}^*} \tag{5}$$

In this context, nobody was so far able to validate whether the elastic modulus of a pharmaceutical compact can be described *by Eq. (5) with the universal critical exponent*

Tablet X Form	Rel. Dens. (L)	TD_{is} (L) (sec)	Predicted Result (sec)	Tablet X Form	Rel Dens. (R)	TD_{is} (R) (sec)	Predicted Result (sec)
D*	*0.818*	—	*789*	F	0.842	266	284
D*'	*0.820*	—	*593*	F'	0.8435	359.5	387
E*	*0.824*	—	*284*	G	0.845	453	505
E*'	*0.836*	—	*31*	G'	0.8465	605.5	639
F	0.842	266	284	H	0.848	758	789

Experimental and predicted results based on Eq. (1). The predicted disintegration time values for the tablets D, D*' E* and E*'correspond* to lower relative densities *of the tablets D, D', E, and E'.*

Table 4.
Data from [10], in blue = interpolated, in red = extrapolated value.

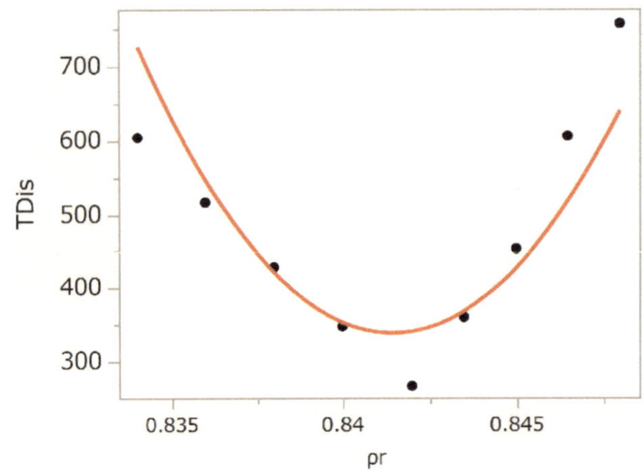

Figure 5.
Non-linear regression analysis for the disintegration time (Y-axis in sec) TDis =7,031,096 (ρ_r, −0.84144)^2 + 338 as a function of the relative density ρ_r, (X-axis = apparent density/real density = relative density). Predicted values of the disintegration time TD_{is} as a function of the relative densities ρ_r of the tablets D, D', E, E', D, D*' E* E*' and F, F', G, G' and H (see* ***Table 5****).*

q = 3.75* [18] and with p = relative density of the compact, respectively, p_c = critical relative density.

Please note that this *universal* critical exponent consists of a *fractal* showing the connection to Mandelbrot's Fractal world [19]. The latter is related to a non-linear relationship of the variables involved. On the other hand, according to the basic percolation theory of Eq. (1), the compactibility [20] of a pharmaceutical powder system is indirectly proportional to the site percolation threshold of the particles of the substances (active pharmaceutical ingredient, excipient).

A soft, plastic material such as PVP shows a low value of the site percolation, and a brittle material such as Emcompress (calcium hydrogen phosphate dihydrate) shows a high value of the site percolation threshold! In the extreme case, that is, if the compactibility is zero, the site percolation threshold corresponds to the relative

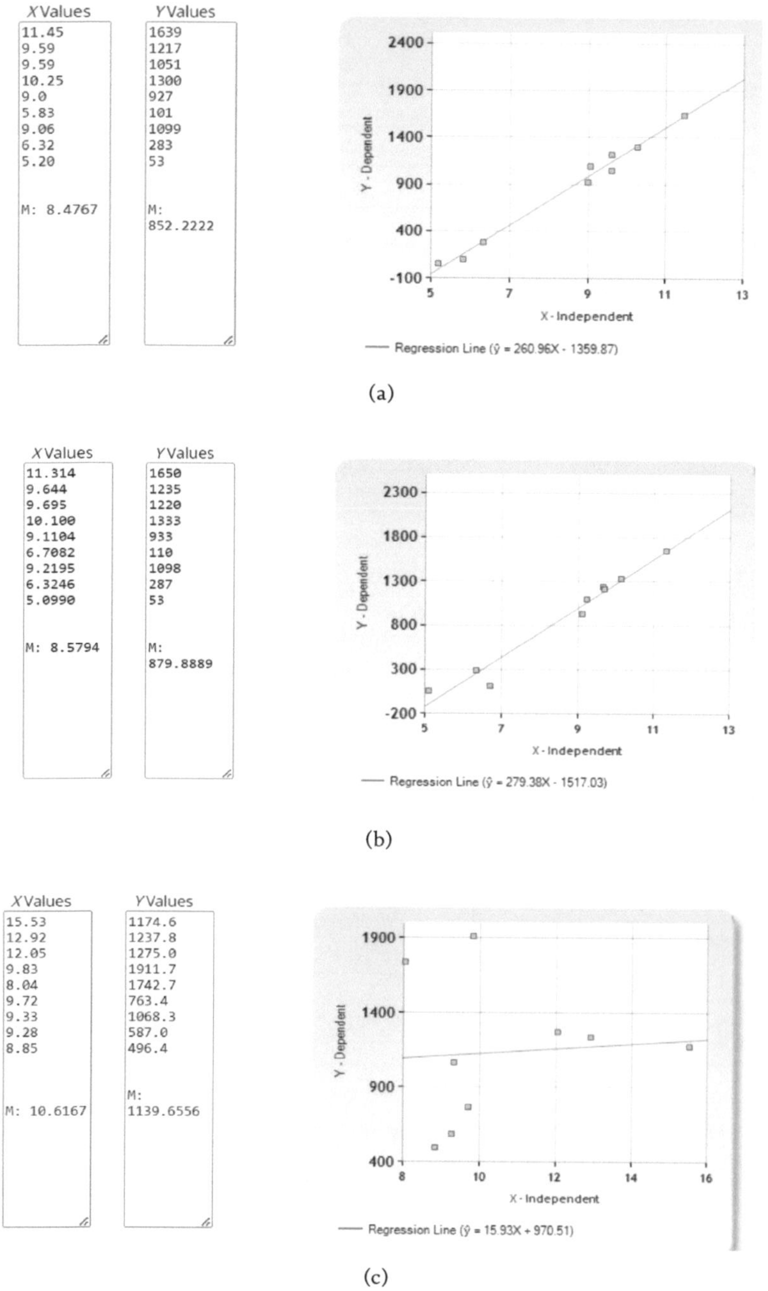

Figure 6.
(a) Correlation between the disintegration time (Y) of the nine nifedipine tablet formulations and the Sqr of the tablet hardness values (X), data from [22], according to ***Table 7****. (b) Validation of the results of* ***Figure 6a*** *by the contract research organization MOAT (X-axis: Sqr [Hardness in N] (****Table 8****), Y-axis: disintegration time in sec).* ***Table 9*** *shows the predicted results of the disintegration tie of the nine nifedipine tablet formulations based on the equation. (c) Unfortunately, no correlation between the disintegration time values (Y) and the square root of the hardness values (X) can be detected. In this context, it needs to be noticed that the addition of approximately 0.05% Magnesium Stearate ("swatch" mixed in a bag) was sufficient to destroy the observed correlation between the critical tablet attribute "disintegration time" and the Sqr of the critical tablet attribute "Hardness". This is a dramatic effect.*

Tablet X Form	Rel. Dens. (L)	TD_{is} (L) (sec)	Predicted Result (sec)	Tablet X Form	Rel Dens. (R)	TD_{is} (R) (sec)	Predicted Result (sec)
D	0.834	604	96	F	0.842	266	0.0
D′	0.836	516	54	F′	0.8435	359.5	3.4
E	0.838	428	24	G	0.845	453	13.5
E'	0.840	347	6.0	G'	0.8465	605.5	30
F	0.842	266	0.0	H	0.848	758	54

Table 5.
Model showing the results for ρ_c = 0.842 with the scaling factor SF = $(1222.8)^2$ according to Eq. (3).

	Composition (% v/v)			MS/(MS + MA)	Disintegration time (sec.)	
	MA	LA	MS		Experimental data (n = 3)	F-CAD data (n = 6)
B	12.0	61.4	26.6	0.698	596 ± 8	338 ± 10
C	23.5	53.4	23.1	0.497	616 ± 6	408 ± 7
D	34.5	45.7	19.8	0.365	604 ± 21	448 ± 14
E	45.0	38.4	16.6	0.27	428 ± 16	395 ± 14
F	55.1	31.3	13.6	0.198	266 ± 8	191 ± 13
G	64.8	24.6	10.6	0.141	453 ± 24	432 ± 19
H	74.1	18.1	7.8	0.096	758 ± 15	785 ± 24
J	34.5	51.3	14.2	0.292	535 ± 12	382 ± 10
K	74.1	12.9	13.0	0.15	413 ± 8	596 ± 9
M	74.0	7.7	18.3	0.198	290 ± 2	897 ± 8
O	34.5	57.0	8.5	0.198	420 ± 9	350 ± 13

The disintegration time predicted by F-CAD corresponds to the calculated time elapsed that the water molecules reach the center of the tablet [16].

Table 6.
Experimental and F-CAD predicted disintegration time of mefenamic acid [MA] tablets [12] consisting of MA, lactose (LA) and maize starch (MS).

density = 1 = zero porosity. In other words, zero compactibility means that there is no bonding between the particles. Thus, due to the lack of bonding, a disordered particulate system may show compressibility = volume reduction under pressure [20] but does not form a stable compact.

A detailed study of an earlier work [21] on the topic of the critical tablet quality attributes, hardness and disintegration time of nifedipine tablet formulations (see **Table 7** and **Figure 6a, b**) showed a correlation between the disintegration time and the hardness of the tablets. *However, this correlation only could be validated for the case that all data (hardness and disintegration) was collected in strict compliance with preparing the tablets by using the original Presster equipment [21] by lubricating the punches and the dies with cotton swabs impregnated with magnesium stearate* instead of mixing the

Disintegration time of Nifedipine tablets at 108,000 TPH, each value represents the mean ± SD (n = 3). Runs according to Table 2					
No.	**Weight (mg)**	**Thickness (mm)**	**Diameter (mm)**	**Hardness (N)**	**Disintegrationtime (sec)**
1	402.7 ± 0.9	4.76 ± 0.02	10.06 ± 0.01	131 ± 13	1639 ± 76
2	401.1 ± 2.0	4.81 ± 0.06	10.08 ± 0.01	92 ± 28	1217 ± 242
3	401.3 ± 0.7	4.76 ± 0.02	10.07 ± 0.01	92 ± 4	1051 ± 348
4	401.0 ± 1.8	4.81 ± 0.06	10.07 ± 0.00	101 ± 12	1300 ± 227
5	401.7 ± 1.0	4.79 ± 0.03	10.08 ± 0.01	81 ± 9	927 ± 43
6	400.2 ± 1.0	4.83 ± 0.03	10.11 ± 0.02	34 ± 18	101 ± 17
7	401.0 ± 1.3	4.85 ± 0.04	10.09 ± 0.00	82 ± 14	1099 ± 20
8	401.5 ± 2.0	4.89 ± 0.03	10.12 ± 0.01	40 ± 7	283 ± 48
9	401.2 ± 0.7	4.86 ± 0.03	10.12 ± 0.01	27 ± 6	53 ± 11

Table 7.
This table corresponds to Table A1b of publication [21] by Duangmanee Maneerojpakdee et al. An attempt to adopt the workflow of the automotive and aircraft industry for the design of drug delivery vehicles.

lubricant (2.0% w/w) with powder particles. In addition, the critical tablet quality attributes need to be measured after 24-hour relaxation of the thermodynamic system, initially far from equilibrium conditions.

$$\text{Disintegration Time} = 279\ \text{Sqr}\ (\text{Hardness}) – 1517\ [\text{sec}] \tag{6}$$

Interestingly, the correlation between the hardness or tensile strength of the nifedipine tablet formulations of **Figure 6a, b**, as well as the successful validation of **Figure 6a**, vanishes if the lubricant Magnesium Stearate is classically distributed in the powder mixture before tableting, as shown in **Figure 6c**.

Indeed, this result corresponds to a fundamental textbook experiment showing the importance of the bonding between the particles in the tablet. This result confirms the interpretation of results obtained in binary powder systems regarding the tensile strength of a tablet [15, 23]. In the case of a binary system, percolation theory was used with a universal critical exponent q^* = 2.7 instead of q^* = 3.75. The interpretation [23] showed the importance of the bonding strength distribution of local bonds between the particles. Thus, it makes sense that the distribution of the hydrophobic lubricant Magnesium Stearate is influencing the bonding capacity, which is mainly based hydrophilic, van der Waals forces. *Thus, the need of an external lubrication device or a hydrophilic lubricant would be advantageous.*

Interestingly, the results of **Figure 6c** could be confirmed in the PhD thesis of Dr. Go Kimura [10]. He also used the Presster equipment for manufacturing the mefenamic acid (MA) tablet formulations and added 0.5% w/w magnesium stearate to the tableting mixture. For this reason, he might not be able to find a correlation between the disintegration time of MA tablet formulations and the Sqr of the tensile strength of the tablets (**Figure 7**), according to **Table 10**.

3.3 "Organic" life, and the regeneration of liver tissue

It is well known that lizards can regenerate tails being damaged. This process is called autotomy [24]. Human beings can regenerate part of the liver after surgery. The

Tablet form	Weight (mg) ± SD (mg)	Thickness ± SD (mm)	Hardness ± SD (N)	Disint. T. ± SD (sec)
Nr 1	397 ± 8	4.0 ± 0.1	128 ± 11	1650 ± 087
Nr 2	401 ± 6	4.0 ± 0.1	93 ± 24	1235 ± 214
Nr 3	402 ± 5	4.0 ± 0.1	94 ± 04	1220 ± 076
Nr 4	400 ± 6	4.1 ± 0.1	102 ± 08	1333 ± 104
Nr 5	401 ± 6	4.0 ± 0.1	84 ± 08	0933 ± 043
Nr 6	396 ± 5	4.0 ± 0.1	45 ± 06	0110 ± 013
Nr 7	400 ± 5	4.0 ± 0.1	85 ± 11	1198 ± 025
Nr 8	399 ± 7	4.0 ± 0.1	40 ± 05	0287 ± 033
Nr 9	400 ± 5	4.0 ± 0.1	26 ± 04	053 ± 011

Table 8.
Validation results of the physical characterization of the nine nifedipine tablet formulations of ***Table** 7* *by CRO MOAT.*

Tablet nifedipine formulation	Rel. Dens	TDis (sec)	Predicted Result (sec) Eq. (3)	Predicted Result (sec) Eq. (4)	Predicted Result (sec) Eq. (6)
1	0.73395	1650	886	926	1640
2	0.73013	1235	946	1047	1174
3	0.76114	1220	308		1188
4	0.69291	1333	1047		1300
5	0.72468	933	1034	1234	1025
6	0.76755	110	444	180	355
7	0.75917	1098	540		1055
8	0.79110	287	224		248
9	0.79001	53.0	233	4	−94.0

In the case of Eq. (3) the predicted values correspond to the following parameters Scaling Factor SF = 66925.7 and critical relative density p_c = 0.849. In the case of Eq. (4) the predicted values correspond to the following parameters Scaling Factor SF = 256744.9 and critical relative density p_c = 0.794. It is important to note that in the case of Eq. (4), only the relevant relative density values were used, as in the case of the mefenamic acid (MA) tablet formulations [10] of the PhD thesis of Dr. Kimura. Due to the range of relative densities studied of the nifedipine tablet formulations, only the left branch of the quadratic function could be studied leading, as expected, to a better prediction of the critical quality attribute "disintegration time" and of the value of the percolation threshold p_c = 0.794 compared to Eq. (3), which is an approximation.

Table 9.
Measured and predicted disintegration times of the nine nifedipine tablet formulations based on Eq. (6) and on assuming that the disintegration time can be described by the basic percolation Eq. (1).

regeneration of liver tissue is very complex and involves many steps of cellular and chemical pathways [25].

In other words, the quality attribute "Liver" as an organ cannot be described by the simple basic percolation Eq. (1) with an appropriate universal exponent q* and a percolation threshold. On the other hand, the quality attribute "liver tissue" is an ordered structure of specific liver cells like the ordered powder particles of a tablet leading to a specific elastic modulus f in the case of "inorganic" life. Thus, in principle,

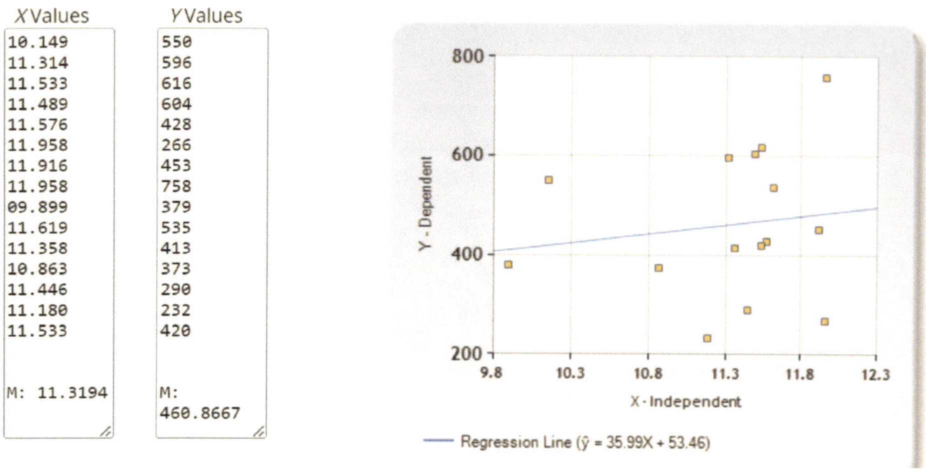

Figure 7.
No correlation between the disintegration time in sec (Y-values) and the Sqr of tensile strength (X-values) of MA tablet formulations could be detected, confirming the results of ***Figure 6c****. This result prompts the idea to manufacture a second set of MA tablet formulations by adding the lubricant externally to evaluate whether the correlation between the critical quality attribute "disintegration time" and the square root of the critical quality attribute "tablet hardness" or "tensile strength" can be validated. Such a validation would be an essential contribution to the concept of quality by design.*

Composition (% v/v)				**MS/MA**		**7 kN**	
					Porosity (% v/v) (n = 6–7)	**TS (N/cm^2) (n = 6–7)**	**TDis (sec.) (n = 3)**
	MA	LA	MS		(n = 6–7)	(n = 6–7)	(n = 3)
A	0	69.7	30.3	—	20.6 ± 0.32	103 ± 3.20	550 ± 23
B	12	61.4	26.6	2.217	18.2 ± 0.21	128 ± 4.64	596 ± 8
C	23.5	53.4	23.1	0.983	17.0 ± 0.28	133 ± 3.60	616 ± 6
D	34.5	45.7	19.8	0.574	16.6 ± 0.28	132 ± 3.89	604 ± 21
E	45.0	38.4	16.6	0.369	16.2 ± 0.20	134 ± 3.35	428 ± 16
F	55.1	31.3	13.6	0.247	15.8 ± 0.24	143 ± 7.14	266 ± 8
G	64.8	24.6	10.6	0.164	15.5 ± 0.14	142 ± 4.76	453 ± 24
H	74.1	18.1	7.8	0.105	16.4 ± 0.37	143 ± 3.52	758 ± 15
I	0	84.8	15.2	—	20.6 ± 0.16	97.6 ± 2.71	379 ± 7
J	34.5	51.3	14.2	0.412	17.0 ± 0.26	135 ± 2.10	536 ± 12
K	74.1	12.9	13.0	0.175	16.3 ± 0.32	129 ± 1.95	413 ± 8
L	0	78.8	21.2	—	19.7 ± 0.15	118 ± 1.96	373 ± 36
M	74.0	7.7	18.3	0.247	16.2 ± 0.11	131 ± 2.17	290 ± 2
N	0	90.9	9.1	—	20.4 ± 0.47	125 ± 4.07	232 ± 20
O	34.5	57.0	8.5	0.246	17.4 ± 0.29	133 ± 4.58	420 ± 9

Table 10.
Excerpt of Table 23 of [10] with list of disintegration time and tensile strength values of mefenamic acid (MA) tablet formulations manufactured with the Presster equipment using a compression force of 7 kN [10].

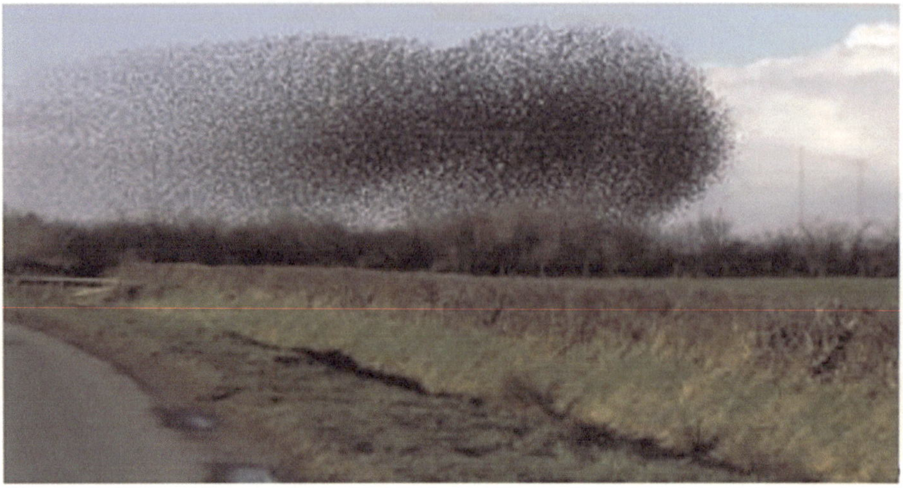

Figure 8.
Flocking of birds [7], Ref Wiki commons.

it can be expected that the basic percolation equation can be used for the description of the ideal volume of the regenerated human liver:

$$\text{Ideal volume of the liver } V_L = SK\left(p\text{–}p_c\right)^{q^*} \qquad (7)$$

with p = density of the human liver cells, p_c = critical density of human liver cells. Indeed, if too much of the liver is removed the liver cannot be reconstituted [25]. Eq. (6) needs to be validated.

The following additional question needs to be addressed: *Do we take care of all cell-to- cell communications, including the possibility of a non-chemical communication, which seems to take place in case of the flocking of birds* (**Figure 8**) [8, 26].

Interestingly, the mechanism of collective "mind change of flying birds" (**Figure 8**) is like a cooperative reaction path of a crystalline phase transition, supporting the idea that similar physical laws exist in "inorganic" and "organic life" [7].

Indeed, the result of the crystallization process leads to a higher order, which can be interpreted as "inorganic life" [7].

The crystalline phase transition keeps a specific order of the system. It can be assumed that the crystallization process can be described by the basic percolation equation with an appropriate exponent.

Thus, the following question arises: Are the current models of a virtual human being complete?

4. The University of Florida College of pharmacy interpretation of life-sciences

Einstein was not sure whether the Copenhagen model of quantum mechanics was complete, known as Copenhagen interpretation [13], sparking the Bohr-Einstein debates [27]. The term Copenhagen "Interpretation" is somehow misleading. In fact, the term "Copenhagen Agreement" between the founding members of the mathematical tools used in quantum mechanics [13] which would be more appropriate.

In this context, Herbert Fröhlich [28] discusses in his chapter "Theoretical Physics and Biology" the problem of cancer in a multicomponent biological system. Fröhlich defines cancer as a transition from an ordered to a disordered state. In other words, Froehlich is convinced that individual cells are subject to a coherent electric vibration of an Einstein-Debye model of cells represented by as system of harmonic oscillators. Thus, a coherent electric vibration extends through the whole tissue (organ), and the vibration of each individual cell responds to it, that is, each cell is held in an appropriate phase and vibrational frequency. Now in cancer, the control exerted by the excited mode is no longer active leading to a phase transition from order to disorder. According to Fröhlich [28] *the disordered (cancer) state, order may be restored by external irradiation with the correct frequency*. Interestingly, the natural personal frequency emitted by late Nishino-sensei was used to treat cancer patients [26]. This fact should promote an intensive study of unresolved mysteries in the manuscript submitted [29]. Interestingly,

Fröhlich's hypothesis opens a new research avenue for the pharmaceutical industry: Can a pharmaceutical active ingredient such as an anti-cancer drug be replaced by an appropriate electromagnetic-acoustic radiation for healing the cancer, respectively restoring the former "higher order" of the system? This idea would comply with the model of the human supercomputer and its architecture needing a control "refreshment cycle" that no important information gets lost.

In this context, the human being is considered as an Einstein-Debye model [30] consisting of harmonic oscillators. These oscillators can be in resonance with water explaining the successful search of talented dowsers. Some dowsers also seem to be sensitive to deposits of silver and gold by holding a piece of silver or gold.

In other words, these findings lead to the surprising hypothesis that the placebo effect could be interpreted as a resonance phenomenon of a specific drug structure. This idea was proposed by Dr. Karim [31], co-chair of the Leuenberger International Symposium on Pharmaceutical Sciences and Processes [32].

This idea prompts the question of whether the "placebo effect" of existing drugs can be reinforced by applying the corresponding electromagnetic-acoustic frequency of the pharmaceutical active ingredient?

Thus, the following hypothesis should be tested: Can we characterize a typical chemical structure such as acetylsalicylic acid, a nonsteroidal anti-inflammatory drug used as a pain killer showing a "placebo effect' of approximately 70%? Can this placebo effect be reinforced by irradiating the patient with drug-typical electromagnetic harmonic and acoustic waves as part of an Einstein-Debye model of Aspirin?

In this context, is the vibrational frequency (infrared frequency) of Aspirin part of the Debey model of the human being? Can such a resonance be detected?

This hypothesis needs to be validated. Irving Kirsch [33], Harvard Medical School, a leading researcher in the field of placebo studies, reported that *antidepressants show a placebo effect close to 80%*. Thus, a second example could be imipramine hydrochloride, a tricyclic antidepressant [34]. The drug's vibrational spectra are known to agree with calculations based on density functional theory [34]. In both examples, it would be important to identify the human Einstein-Debye electromagnetic and acoustic frequencies and the expected resonance with the crystalline structures of the drugs.

5. Conclusions

The basic equation of percolation theory can describe a critical quality attribute such as the disintegration time showing a higher order of the system, respectively, a lower entropy. This property was coined "Inorganic Life" [7] since formulations often also include inorganic components. The main point is the limited number of building blocks, respectively, and the limited degree of freedom in inorganic chemistry compared to organic chemistry leading to a limited number of systems of higher order such as crystals. We know 32 crystal classes, and 7 crystal systems, triclinic, monoclinic, orthorhombic, tetragonal, trigonal, hexagonal and cubic. The "alphabet" of "organic life", that is, the DNA building blocks, leads to the description of the highest order and the highest degree of freedom, respectively, to a large variability of life in our organic ecosystem.

The inorganic life of the critical quality attribute "disintegration time" can be described by the universal critical exponent $q^* = 2$ of Eq. (1).

It was not possible to show the exact value of the universal critical exponent q^* in case of the critical quality attribute "Hardness", "Elastic Modulus" or "Tensile Strength" of a pharmaceutical formulation. This fact may be because usually a hydrophobic lubricant is added to a pharmaceutical formulation, leading to a change in the bonding of the particles involved and to a decrease in the order of the system, respectively in an increase of disorder or entropy (**Figures 4** and **6c**).

Thus, according to the result of the empirical relationship of Eq. (6), it can be assumed in a first approximation that the critical tablet quality attribute for the "Hardness" H is proportional to the critical tablet quality attribute $(TDis)^2$.

Thus, the critical exponent for the critical tablet quality attribute Hardness H is expected to be $q^* = 4$ being close to $q^* = 3.75$. On the other hand, we know that Hardness values are proportional to the values of the deformation hardness and Young's Elastic Modulus according to the work of Sun et al. [17]. This fact prompts the question, whether $q^* = 3.75$ or $q^* = 4.0$ corresponds to the *universal* critical exponent for the Elastic Modulus since an earlier study by Martin Kuentz [35] showed $q^* = 3.95 \pm 0.14$ for Microcrystalline Cellulose (MCC). In other words, to be on the safe side, a third formulation system different from nifedipine and MCC needs to be tested that the *universal* critical exponent $q^* = 4.00$ for Young's Modulus and not $q^* = 3.75$ [18].

Fröhlich [28] describes in his book that human beings are sensitive to electromagnetic smog developing an allergy. On the other hand, he defines "cancer" as a transition from a higher order to a disorder, which can be restored by irradiating the human being with the appropriate electromagnetic radiation. *This hypothesis opens a new research avenue which needs to be explored in detail.*

At the same time his hypothesis supports the idea that the human being can be described as a supercomputer architecture which needs a wireless cell-to-cell communication, like the communication between flocking of birds [7, 36] that no information = order get lost. In this context, it makes sense to explore in more detail the radiation emitted by the followers of the Nishino Breathing method [7, 29, 37–39].

As already mentioned in [7], the human supercomputer as Virtual Patient opens new research avenues with respect to combination products of already registered low-dose safe generic formulations with the advantage that the number of necessary animals and preclinical trials can be reduced with the goal to detect new medical therapies with less side effects.

Contrary to the Copenhagen Interpretation or Agreement, there is no special need to create a different set of mathematical equations like the Schrödinger or Dirac equation since Prigogine and Nicolis provide us with the appropriate mathematical tools and new laws to describe biological phenomena such as the heartbeat regulation [40].

In the above-mentioned proposal of the University of Florida College of Pharmacy Interpretation of Life-Sciences, it is important to complement the new laws of Nobel Laureate Prigogine with *additional simple equations describing the bottom-up principle from simple to complex,* inspired by the ideas of Benoit Mandelbrot [19], Herbert Fröhlich [28], Dieter Stauffer and Amnon Aharoni [9].

In other words, such an approach corresponds to the contrary of reductionism [35], respectively, of a reductionistic method. Thus, percolation theory and its bridge to the fractal nature of Mandelbrot's world [9, 19] may lead to new insights. Fröhlich [28] also suggests studying non-linear systems with the capability to explain more complex biological systems starting from a simpler description.

In other words, according to Prigogine and Nicolis [5–7, 40] new laws related to chaos theory and to non-linear systems need to be considered.

In this context, let us invite the scientific community and the interested members of the University of Florida Center of Pharmacometrics and Systems Pharmacology (CPSP) to explore complex systems in a "bottom up" instead of a reductionistic "top down" approach by promoting the concept of the University of Florida College of Pharmacy Interpretation of Life-Sciences.

As mentioned in the introduction, the model of a virtual patient described as a human supercomputer needs additional improvements that can be provided by modern tools of artificial intelligence, such as deep learning etc. Additional expertise from the part of the computer architecture of commercially available high-speed computers is welcome.

This scientific approach can lead to new insights and hopefully resolve problems by reducing side effects such as the application of "friendly viral infections" attacking only antibiotic-resistant bugs, as "phage" therapy [41] or in the treatment of cancer cells using "phage" therapy as the only food for such "friendly" viral infections. In this context, in the PhD thesis of Dr. Matthias Plitzko, respectively, the Meridion technology [42] for manufacturing nanoparticulate formulations based on the spray-freeze drying technology may be helpful.

It is important to notice that we work in an open thermodynamic system with an influx of energy far from equilibrium conditions, which is an advantage. Thus, the effect of the type of energy input as food also plays an important role. In this context, knowledge of Chinese nutrition therapy [43] can lead to additional insights.

It is well known that in the case of a closed system without influx of energy, the second law of thermodynamics leads to an increase in entropy and disorder. This fact allows us to calculate the expiry date of a pharmaceutical tablet containing a minimum of 90% of pharmaceutical ingredient(s).

For this purpose, the Arrhenius equation often is used to describe the degradation rate $k = A\ e^{-Ea/kT}$ with activation energy:

$$\text{Degradation rate } k = A\ e^{-Ea/RT} \tag{8}$$

with E_a = activation energy.

In addition to the statement that the basic equation of the percolation theory inherently describes a higher order of a system, the following question arises: Can we postulate a regeneration rate constant k* for a regeneration process, reducing the entropy,

$$k^* == A^*\ e^{-E(L)/RT} \tag{9}$$

with E(L) = Life energy of an open thermodynamic system far from equilibrium conditions?

Is it possible to quantitatively determine this energy E(L), which is often called "KI" [8]. that is, "life" energy in the Asian culture?

Can this energy explain the incredible findings of Marcel Violet [8] that his "gold" water is promoting the growth of potatoes and carrots [29, 43]?

In both cases [7, 8], the "life energy" is of electromagnetic nature.

In other words, it can be assumed that Marcel Violet's process to obtain his "gold" water induced an "Anderson" localization of electromagnetic energy [8], which was stored for a limited time and subsequently consumed by the biological system, leading to a better crop. This hypothesis needs to be validated.

Interestingly, Comunetti [8] could confirm the results of the "Anderson" localization of electromagnetic waves in the range of electromagnetic energies of gamma rays capable of inducing a photo-nuclear reaction which can be used to treat radioactive waste of nuclear power plants to remove the radioactivity of the waste.

On the other hand, the corresponding author was tempted not to publish the work of Dr. Angelo Comunetti, since his method can be used to develop powerful gamma lasers.

Most important is the fact that the "Anderson" localization accumulated electromagnetic energy that was consumed by the cells of Marcel Violet's biological system fertilizing carrots and potatoes and can be used for avoiding pollution of the environment with artificial fertilizers such as urea and phosphate.

Interestingly, in the case of Marcel Violet's experiments, no chemical energy was involved as in the case of "flocking" of birds [7, 36].

On the other hand, in principle, E(L) does not need to be of electromagnetic nature but could be of chemical nature in the open thermodynamic system.

Thus, it would be of interest to know whether E(L) also is a function of the energy input, that is, of food [44]?

In other words, food, lifestyle and the appropriate ethical codex are important factors for a sustainable health and peaceful society.

Acknowledgements

The corresponding author thanks Prof. Sarah Kim, University of Florida, College of Pharmacy, for her initial proposal to include interested members of the Center of Pharmacometrics and Systems Pharmacology of the Orlando Campus, as co-authors of the book chapter. It is a pity that Sarah did not have additional time to contribute with her skills to the contents of the book chapter. Dr. Michael Levin, and Ofer Aqua, CRO MOAT Advanced Technologies, thank Prof Stephan Schmidt for the financial contribution from the College of Pharmacy of the University of Florida and from the company IFIIP, Institute for Innovation in Industrial Pharmacy, Orlando, allowing to support the experimental work. At the same time, all authors acknowledge the company Pharmatrans Sanaq, Allschwil, Switzerland, for supporting the project of the book chapter with the excipients needed.

In addition, the corresponding author thanks Dr. Florian Kongoli, President of SIPS for inviting him to organize in his name the Leuenberger International Symposium on Sustainable Pharmaceutical Sciences and Industrial Applications for Sustainable Development. In this context, Hans Leuenberger thanks Prof Marcel Tanner, former President of the Swiss Academies of Arts and Sciences for supporting the idea of the symposium and especially thanks his former PhD students, Prof Georgios Imanidis, Dr. Stephan Buchmann, Dr. Go Kimura, Dr. Matthias Plitzko, Dr. Hassan Tarabishi, Dr. Andreas Tschirky, and his friends Dr. Martin Bultmann, Dr. Leo Eskin, Engineer Francois Comunetti, son of Dr. Angelo Comunetti, Markus H Jordi-Koi, Dr. Ibrahim Karim, Dr. Maria Olga Kokornaczyk, Prof Natalia Menshutina, Daniel R

Salazar Montero, Dr. Norbert and Julius Schwarzer, Hiba Tarabishi, Prof Vincenz von Tscharner, Heather van Wolf and Markus Jordi, Prof Albert Winkler for presenting lectures at the Leuenberger symposium of the 2024 SIPS summit, October 20–24, in Crete, Greece.

The presentations included transdisciplinary lectures promoting fair trade in goldmining, green agriculture and biogeometry research results. The quest for a scientific explanation of water dowsing and sustainability in big pharma – Can supercomputer do the magic? Formulation development of co-crystal compound in Shionogi; Promoting innovation efforts; Sustainability in medicine and pharmaceutics – what can we learn from history? Aseptic spray freeze drying, the impact of structured water; Aerogels – new delivery systems, modeling, Ethical history – a contradiction in terms? What are the effects of conflict on supply chains and trade within the pharmaceutical industry: The case of Syria; A fast method to detect the efficiency of antibiotic treatment in case of sepsis; open-mindedness and unresolved mysteries (in pharmaceutical sciences). The contribution "Love, the black hole in the universe of feelings – why psychology might need quantum gravity concepts" complemented the contribution "The legacy of the Swiss hermit Nicolas of Flue leading to the World Health Organization (WHO) Peace Initiative".

The authors thank Dr. Shukla, Academic Editor, for his recommendations to optimize the contents of the book chapter. The corresponding author thanks the following persons for fruitful discussions Marcel Duerrenberger, Dan Lionberger, Philippe Comunetti, Hassan Tarabishi , Randy Hardy, Ted Mann, Daniel Salazar, Peter Swaan, Elena O'Keeff and Susanna Rehmann.

Author details

Hans Leuenberger[1*], Stephan Schmidt[1], Go Kimura[2], Michael Levin[3] and Ofer Aqua[3]

1 Department of Pharmaceutics, Center for Pharmacometrics and Systems Pharmacology, College of Pharmacy, University of Florida, Orlando, FL, USA

2 Formulation R&D Laboratory, CMC Research Innovation Center, Shionogi & Co., Ltd, Amagasaki, Japan

3 CRO MOAT, c/o Ofer Aqua, Ofer Aqua, Ofra, Israel

*Address all correspondence to: hans.leuenberger@cop.ufl.edu

References

[1] Schmidt S, Vozmediano V, Cristofoletti R, et al. Requirements, expectations, challenges and opportunities associated with training the next generation of pharmacometricians. CPT: Pharmacometrics & Systems Pharmacology. 2023;**12**:883-888. DOI: 10.1002/psp4.1297021638306, 2023, 7

[2] College of Pharmacy at the University of Florida [Internet]. Available from: https://pharmacy.ufl.edu/the-college/faculty-staff/

[3] Center of Pharmacometrics and Systems Pharmacology of the College of Pharmacy at the University of Florida [Internet]. Available from: https://expertnet.org/index.cfm?fuseaction=centers.details&instituteID=5632

[4] University of Florida, College of Pharmacy Winter School [Internet]. Available from: https://pharmacy.ufl.edu/florida-winter-school/

[5] Prigogine I, Stengers I. Order out of Chaos. London, New York: Verso; 2017. pp. 1-349

[6] Prigogine I. The End of Certainty, Time, Chaos, and the New Laws of Nature. New York: The Free Press; 1997. pp. 1-227

[7] Leuenberger H. The organic supercomputer able to replicate, as virtual patient. In: Kongoli F, Murad F, Yoshikawa T, Ribas JR, Joseph D, Tran N, Hirano S, editors. 2023 SIPS Proceedings, Panama, Proceedings of 2023 Sustainable Industrial Processing Summit. Vol. 11. FLOGEN; 2023

[8] Comunetti AM, Leuenberger H. Lockage of the first excited stage of ^{198}Hg. In: Kongoli F, Murad F, Yoshikawa T, Ribas JR, Joseph D, Tran N, Hirano S, editors. Proceedings of 2023 Sustainable Industrial Processing Summit. Vol. 11. FLOGEN; 2023

[9] Stauffer D, Aharony A. Introduction to Percolation Theory. 2nd ed. London, Bristol (USA): Taylor and Francis; 1994. pp. 1-181

[10] Kimura G. Design of pharmaceutical tablet formulations for a low water-soluble drug: search for the critical concentration of starch base disintegrant applying percolation theory and F-CAD (formulation – computer aided design) [thesis]. Switzerland: Faculty of Science, University of Basel; 2012

[11] F-CAD (Formulation- Computer Aided Design) by CINCAP [Internet]. Available from: https://www.f-cad.ch/

[12] Luginbuehl R, Leuenberger H. Use of percolation theory to interpret water uptake, disintegration time and intrinsic dissolution rate of tablets consisting of binary mixtures. Pharmaceutica Acta Helvetia. 1994;**69**:127-134

[13] Kopenhagen Interpretation [Internet]. Available from: https://en.wikipedia.org/wiki/Copenhagen_interpretation

[14] T'Hooft G. The Cellular Automaton Interpretation of Quantum Mechanics. Springer; 2016. pp. 1-293

[15] Kuentz M, Leuenberger H, Kolb M. Fracture in disordered media and tensile strength of microcrystalline cellulose tablets at low relative densities. International Journal of Pharmaceutics. 1999;**182**:243-255

[16] Leuenberger H, Puchkov M, Schneider B. Right first time concept and workflow. Swiss Pharma. 2013;**35**:3-16

[17] Sun W-J, Kothari S, Sun CC. The relationship among tensile strength (Young's) elastic modulus and indentation hardness of pharmaceutical compacts. Powder Technology. 2018;**331**: 1-6

[18] Leuenberger H. The application of percolation theory in powder technology. Advanced Powder Technology. 1999;**10**:323-352

[19] Mandelbrot B. The Fractal Geometry of Nature. New York: Freeman; 1983. pp. 1-468

[20] Leuenberger H. The compressibility and compactibility of powder systems. International Journal of Pharmaceutics. 1982;**12**:41-55

[21] Maneerojpakdee D et al. An attempt to adopt the workflow of the automotive and aircraft industry for the design of drug delivery vehicles. Pharm Tech Japan. 2017;**33**(11):145-156

[22] Liver regeneration [Internet]. Available from: https://en.wikipedia.org/wiki/Liver_regeneration

[23] Ramírez N et al. Comparison of different mathematical models for the tensile strength–relative density profiles of binary tablets. European Journal of Pharmaceutical Sciences. 2004;**22**:19-23

[24] Autotomy [Internet] Available from: https://en.wikipedia.org/wiki/Autotomy

[25] Huang W, Han N, Du L, Wang M, Chen L, Tang H. A narrative review of liver regeneration—From models to molecular basis. Annals of Translational Medicine. 2021;**9**(22):1705. DOI: 10.21037/atm-21-5234

[26] Nishino-sensei, personal communication.

[27] Bohr-Einstein Debates [Internet]. Available from: https://en.wikipedia.org/wiki/Bohr-Einstein_debates

[28] Froehlich H. Biological Coherence and Response to External Stimuli. Berlin, Heidelberg, New York, London, Paris, Tokyo: Springer; 1988. pp. 1-265

[29] Leuenberger H. Open mindedness and unresolved mysteries. In: Manuscript Uploaded for the 2024 SIPS Leuenberger International Symposium for Sustainable Pharmaceutical Sciences and Processes, Crete, October 20–24. 2024

[30] Einstein Debye Model [Internet]. Available from: https://en.wikipedia.org/wiki/Debye_model

[31] Karim I. personal communication.

[32] Leuenberger International Symposium on sustainable Pharmaceutical Sciences and Processes [Internet]. Available from: https://www.flogen.org/sips2024/Hans_Leuenberger.php

[33] Irving Kirsch [Internet]. Available from: https://en.wikipedia.org/wiki/Irving_Kirsch

[34] Sagdinc SG, Azkeskin C, Esime A. Theoretical and spectroscopic studies of tricyclic antidepressant, imipramine hydrochloride. Journal of Molecular Structure. 2018;**1161**:169-184

[35] Kuentz M, Leuenberger H. Modified Young's modulus of microcrystalline cellulose and the directed continuum percolation model. Pharmaceutical Development and Technology. 1998;**3**: 13-19

[36] Reductionism [Internet]. Available from: https://en.wikipedia.org/wiki/Reductionism

[37] Flocking of Birds [Internet]. Available from: https://en.wikipedia.org/wiki/Flock_(birds)#

[38] Nishino Breathing Method [Internet]. Available from: https://nishinojuku.com/en/

[39] Ohnishi ST, Ohnishi T. The Nishino breathing method and Ki-energy (life energy): A challenge to traditional scientific thinking. Evidence-based Complementary and Alternative Medicine. 2006;**3**(2):191-200. DOI: 10.1093/exam/ne1004, open access

[40] Nicolis G, Prigogine I, Complexity E. Piper. Munich: GmbH & Co. KG; 1989. pp. 1-313

[41] Phage Therapy [Internet]. Available from: https://en.wikipedia.org/wiki/Phage_therapy

[42] Leuenberger H. Spray freeze-drying for formulations of precision medicine & vaccines. Swiss Pharma. 2021;**43**(4): 10-18

[43] Violet M, Remy M. Le Secret des Patriarches 1962 [Internet]. Available from: http://laforceuniverselle.free.fr

[44] Kastner J. Chinese Nutrition Therapy. 2nd ed. Stuttgart, New York: Thieme; 2003. pp. 1-278

Chapter 6

Advancements in Omeprazole Formulations: From Technological Innovation to Release Strategies

Ioanna Papoutsi, Angeliki Siamidi, Nefeli Lagopati, Maria Gazouli, Marilena Vlachou and Natassa Pippa

Abstract

This chapter reviews data on 72 omeprazole (OME) formulations developed in the past 5 years. The types of OME formulations, the excipients and the methods are analyzed in depth. Data on 72 omeprazole (OME) formulations created over the last 5 years are reviewed in this chapter. A thorough analysis of the many kinds of OME formulations, excipients and techniques is conducted. The release of OME from various formulations, the variables influencing this release, and how it affects the efficacy of the medication are also covered in this chapter. The review seeks to identify significant distinctions and parallels between these formulations and their constituent parts by contrasting the data gathered.

Keywords: omeprazole, formulations, drug-delivery systems, sustained release, controlled release, hydrogels, tablets, capsules, nanoformulations, added value, therapeutic value, repurposing

1. Introduction

Omeprazole (OME, **Figure 1a**) and its *S*-isomer, esomeprazole (**Figure 1b**), are potent benzimidazole derivatives and antisecretory drugs, which belong to the widely used group of proton pump inhibitors (PPIs) [1]. OME works by inhibiting the critical enzyme H^+/K^+ ATPase, which is located in the parietal cells of the stomach and is commonly referred as the proton pump. This enzyme plays a crucial role in the final step of gastric acid production, and by inhibiting it, OME effectively reduces gastric acid secretion [2].

Omeprazole's primary indications include the treatment of gastric [3] and duodenal ulcers, prevention of gastric and duodenal ulcers related to the use of nonsteroidal anti-inflammatory drugs (NSAIDs), and prevention of ulcer recurrence. It is also used for the treatment of symptomatic gastroesophageal reflux disease (GERD), esophagitis, Barrett's esophagus and functional dyspepsia. Additionally, omeprazole

IntechOpen

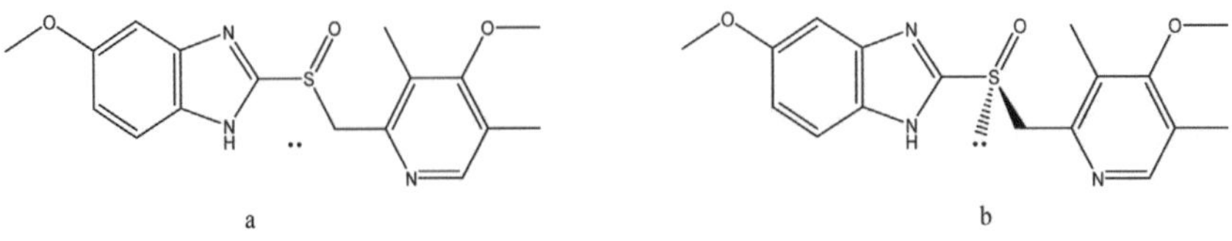

Figure 1.
(a) Chemical structure of omeprazole; (b) chemical structure of esomeprazole.

is a key component in the eradication of *Helicobacter pylori* infections in peptic ulcer disease and in managing complex hypersecretory syndromes, such as the Zollinger-Ellison syndrome [4].

One of the major pharmaceutical challenges with omeprazole, as with other PPIs, is the stability issue. Omeprazole is highly sensitive to the acidic environment and degrades rapidly under the stomach conditions [5]. Thus, its orally administered formulations have to be carefully selected, in order to ensure that OME remains intact, while passing through the stomach and is only released in the small intestine, which typically has a more neutral environment. To overcome this significant issue, omeprazole is usually formulated with the incorporation of an enteric coating, which prevents premature degradation [6]. Alternative delivery systems, such as oral suspensions and intravenous formulations, have also been developed for children and patients who may face specific difficulties, such as cataposis-related problems [7].

In the last 35 years, since its initial launch in Europe in 1988 and its subsequent introduction to the United States market in 1989 under the brand name Prilosec®, developed by Astra AB company (now named Astra Zeneca®) [8], omeprazole formulations have undergone significant advancements. Numerous innovative formulations have been examined, in order to enhance omeprazole's characteristics, in terms of stability, release profile and therapeutic efficacy [9]. Furthermore, in recent years, attempts have been made, to explore OME's full potential and its repurposing profile with respect to other promising therapeutic uses, like cancer treatment [10]. These developments demonstrate not only the drug's long-standing importance in the field of gastroenterology, but also its long-lasting role in pharmaceutical innovation.

2. Omeprazole's formulations over the last 5 years: Literature review

2.1 Methodology

To include as many relevant articles on the topic as possible, a search was conducted, in July 2024, using the electronic database "PubMed" for articles published within the last 5 years.

The search terms were the English words "omeprazole" and "formulation" along with specific keywords, such as "tablets", "capsules", "solid lipid nanoparticles", "hydrogels", "pellets" and "nanogels." The search strategy flowchart was recorded and is illustrated in **Figure 2**.

Initially, articles were excluded from the review based on their titles, as it was being clear that they did not focus on the topic under study. For example, excluded were those, which have dealt with either the therapeutic effects of other active substances or studies involving animal populations.

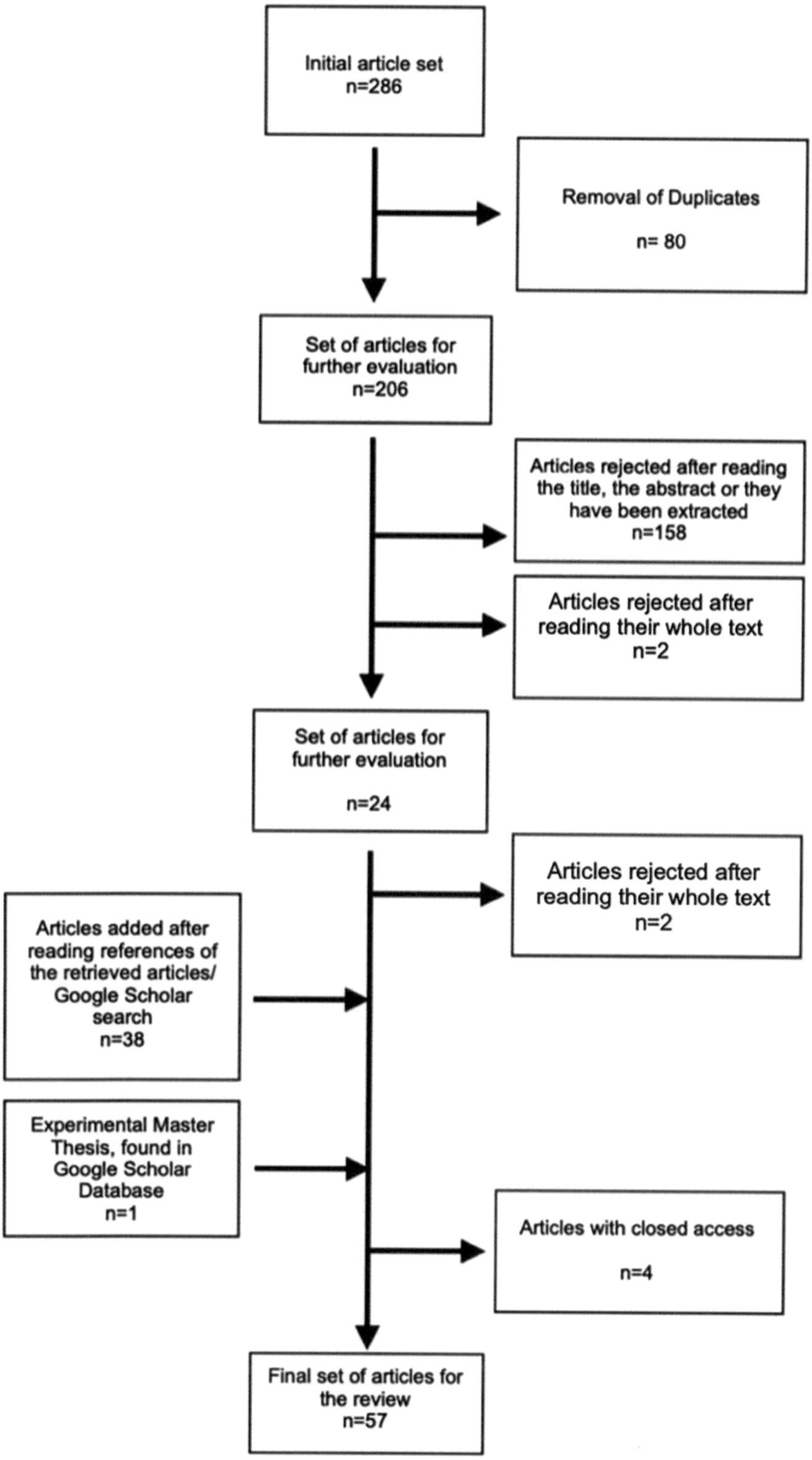

Figure 2.
Search strategy flowchart.

Additionally, articles that reviewed the formulations bibliographically, rather than presenting original research, were also not taken into account.

The number of articles selected for further investigation was n = 22. However, this number was considered insufficient and a second search with the same search terms was conducted in the Google Scholar database. Furthermore, in order to maximize the inclusion of more relevant and appropriate articles the references of the retrieved articles were also examined. To conclude, the final set of articles for the review was n = 57. However, only the optimized formulations mentioned in the articles/studies and/or those with notable characteristics are presented in this review.

Additionally, the pharmaceutical forms are ranked according to decreasing frequency (**Tables 1** and **2**). Frequency tables and graphs about the release type and added value of the formulations are also included.

2.2 Pharmaceutical forms

2.2.1 Solid dosage forms

This chapter overviews various solid dosage forms of omeprazole made in the last 5 years, including tablets, capsules and an oral thin film, each employing distinct methods and excipients to optimize omeprazole delivery and bioavailability. A subchapter follows, overviewing the semi-solid dosage forms, including omeprazole-loaded gels, buccal foams and a suppository.

The study by Mohaparta et al. [11] describes a formulation of delayed-release omeprazole tablets *via* the wet granulation method. The main excipients, lactose monohydrate and sodium starch glycolate, were used in different ratios to prepare the core tablets, which were evaluated for their hardness, thickness, strength and weight variation. The spraying technique was used for sub-coating with hypromellose E5 LV and other excipients in different ratios. Furthermore, different concentrations of enteric coating solutions with HPMC AS MF, triethyl citrate and Opadry brown were

Type of Release	Tablets (22)	Nanoparticles (13)	Liquid formulations (8)	Capsules (6)	Gels (6)
Immediate	5	0	1	1	0
Delayed	4	0	1	2	0
Sustained	6	3	1	0	4
Gradual	1	0	1	0	0
Controlled	4	3	1	3	1
Stable	1	0	0	0	0
Unknown	1	6	2	0	1
Sustained and controlled	0	0	1	0	0
pH depended	0	1	0	0	0

Table 1.
Type of release of the five most frequent formulation types.

Type of release	Total
Immediate	9
Delayed	9
Sustained	16
Gradual	2
Controlled	13
Stable	1
Unknown	12
Sustained and controlled	1
pH depended	1
Extended	1
Rapid	1
Burst	5

Table 2.
Frequency of release types of 71 out of 72 formulations. One formulation (semi-solid printable formulation) did not involve a release study in acidic media and therefore was not measured.

tested *in vitro*, with respect to drug release and acid resistance. When 25% of coating was used, the optimized Batch 2 met the criteria for gastroresistance and showed 97% drug release within 1 h, at pH 6.8. Furthermore, X-ray diffraction (XRD), differential scanning calorimetry (DSC) and Fourier-transform infrared spectroscopy (FTIR) studies revealed the amorphous *versus* crystalline state drug of the drug in the tablet formulation, showing no significant changes after 3 months of accelerated stability testing. Thus, the main advantage of this formulation is its gastroresistance and delayed release.

In another study, the formulation of delayed-release omeprazole sodium tablets was investigated [12]. Direct compression and non-aqueous granulation methods were used to prepare the first two and the second three tablet formulations, respectively, where the excipients mannitol, heavy magnesium oxide, L-HPC-LH 21 and others were used in different ratios. Formulation five batch, which exhibited good flow properties and met quality parameters (appearance, thickness, weight variation, hardness, friability and disintegration time), was selected for sub-coating with Opardy clear and enteric HPMCP coating. *In vitro* dissolution and stability studies identified SE12 (Sub and Enteric-Coated Formulation number 12) as the optimal formulation with a 6% (w/w) sub-coating and 14% (w/w) enteric coating. SE12 showed no significant changes after 3 months of accelerated stability testing. A comparison of assay, drug release, acid resistance and dissolution profile of SE12 with innovator tablet showed no major differences. Consequently, the formulation offers no notable added value.

In a more advanced approach, Trimukhe et al. [13] examined the formulation of delayed-release omeprazole tablets using pulsed radio frequency plasma for the functionalization of omeprazole microparticles with methacrylic acid (MAA) and methyl methacrylate (MMA). The plasma-treated omeprazole powder was compressed into tablets. *In vitro* dissolution studies showed 3.6–9.1% release within 120 minutes, at pH 1.2, *versus* complete release within 60 minutes, at pH 6.8. X-ray photoelectron spectroscopy (XPS) revealed increased oxygen-containing surface groups. Raman analysis indicated no peaks between 1800 and 1000 cm^{-1} in the spectrum, indicating that there were no significant structural changes to the omeprazole's structure due to the plasma treatment. Thermal, nuclear magnetic resonance (NMR) and high-resolution mass spectrometry (HR-MS) analyses also confirmed no alteration of OME's chemical structure through the deposition process, while the decreased contact angle suggested increased surface hydrophilicity. X-ray diffraction showed improved crystallinity and larger crystal size. Scanning electron microscopy (SEM) and dynamic light scattering (DLS) confirmed consistent particle size. Therefore, this formulation provides a safe and cost-effective, alternative drug surface modification method.

On the other hand, attention has also been drawn toward the development of immediate release and fast disintegrating formulations to improve convenience of dosing when quick onset of action is required or when there are cataposis-related problems.

The study by Pavan et al. [14] describes the formulation of immediate-release omeprazole tablets. The excipients microcrystalline cellulose, sodium starch glycolate, lactose anhydrous, the surfactant sodium lauryl sulfate and others were used in varying concentrations to formulate nine different batches *via* the direct compression method. Pre-compression parameters: Carr's index, Hausner's ratio and angle of repose showed good flow properties of the powders. Post-compression parameters: thickness, average weight, hardness, friability, disintegration time, drug content and wetting time were also assessed and showed that all batches passed the pharmacopeia limits. Formulation number 9 with a ratio of 1:1 sodium starch glycolate to sodium lauryl sulfate was selected as the optimized batch, as it was found to have faster wetting ability (6.1 ± 1.1 sec) and higher drug release (98,1% omeprazole release within 60 min) compared to others. Therefore, this formulation offers ease and convenience of dosing.

Additionally, there is a study [15] that describes the formulation of bi-layered tablets for the co-delivery of clarithromycin and instant-release omeprazole as anti-*H. pylori* agents. Nine formulations of omeprazole layer were prepared by direct compression, with a varying ratio of microcrystalline cellulose, croscarmellose sodium, crospovidone and other excipients. Instant release layer formulation number 6 (IF-6) (Croscarmellose sodium: omeprazole = 4:1) was selected as the optimized batch. Accordingly, nine formulations of clarithromycin layer were prepared by direct compression, with a varying ratio of HPMC K 15, HPMC K 4, $NaHCO_3$, lactose and other excipients. Formulation number 8 (HPMC K 15: HPMC K 4: Lactose = 85:85:30) was selected as the optimum batch. Fourier-transform infrared spectroscopy showed no drug-excipient interactions, including the absence of any new peaks indicating chemical bonding, hydrogen bonding or molecular rearrangement. These optimized layers were compressed together into bilayered tablets and evaluated for hardness, friability, weight variation and thickness, all of which were within the acceptable limits. *In vitro* drug release studies showed 99.45% omeprazole release at 15 min and 98.23% clarithromycin release over 12 hours. Hence, this co-delivery system is advantageous because the combination of both drugs enhances therapeutic efficacy against *H. pylori*. Additionally, it improves clarithromycin's bioavailability, simplifies dosing and may lead to better patient compliance in treating *H. pylori* infections. Furthermore, it reduces manufacturing costs.

The study by Srujana et al. [16] investigates the formulation of oral disintegrating omeprazole tablets using the excipients hydroxypropyl beta-cyclodextrin, lactose, mannitol and others, in varying ratios. Nine batches were prepared by the wet granulation method and evaluated for weight variation, hardness, friability, disintegration and *in vitro* dissolution, all meeting the official standards. All tablets disintegrated in less than 60 sec, with the optimized formulation number 1 (lactose: hydroxy propyl beta-cyclodextrin: croscarmellose sodium: hydroxy propyl methyl cellulose = 33:50:21:4 mg) disintegrating in 15 sec and achieving 98.55% drug release at t = 12 hours. Consequently, the added value of this formulation lies in its ease of administration to people with dyscataposis and to children.

Expanding on this concept, the research by Bhamare et al. [17] examined the formulation of fast-disintegrating omeprazole tablets by the direct compression method. Microcrystalline cellulose, mannitol and other excipients were used in varying ratios, preparing nine different batches. Preformulation studies, like bulk density, tapped density angle of repose, Carr's Index and Hauser's ratio, showed that all nine blends met the official standards. The formulated tablets were evaluated for their weight variation, hardness, thickness, friability, disintegration time and *in vitro* drug release. The optimized formulation number 3 (F3), containing 12 mg crospovidone, achieved a 98.38% drug release in 10 seconds, improving the bioavailability of omeprazole through buccal mucosa by bypassing the hepatic first-pass metabolism.

Similarly, another study [18] investigated the formulation of omeprazole mucoadhesive buccal tablets. Nine distinct formulations were prepared by direct compression, using the excipients microcrystalline cellulose, HPMC K4M and sodium alginate, among others, in varying ratios. Fourier-transform infrared spectroscopy confirmed compatibility among drugs and excipients. The powder blends demonstrated within prescribed limits flow properties, making them suitable for tablet compression. Post-compression parameters; weight variation, hardness, thickness, friability, drug content uniformity, surface pH and *in vitro* drug release were evaluated. Batch formulation number 4 (F4) with HPMC K4M: MCC in approximately 1:5 ratio had a drug content of 99,61% and showed the maximum omeprazole release among the formulations: 99,54% over 8 hours at pH 6,8. *In vitro* release kinetics studies showed that F4 follows the Higuchi model. All evaluation parameters met the official standards, suggesting that the mucoadhesive buccal tablets could bypass the hepatic first-pass metabolism, improving the bioavailability of omeprazole through buccal mucosa.

Continuing the modified release/delivery, the study by Kaushal et al. [19] explored the formulation of a floating omeprazole tablet for antacid therapy. The wet granulation method was used to prepare nine omeprazole tablet formulations with a varying ratio of lactose, HPMC K15 and HPMC K100, among other excipients. Fourier-transform infrared spectroscopy and differential scanning calorimetry confirmed no interaction between the drug and the excipients. Formulation number 3 (F3) (HPMC K100:HPMC K15M:lactose = 125:50:210) was selected as the optimized batch, having an *in vitro* drug release of 9.34% in 2 h at pH 1.2 and 91.25% in 24 h at pH 1.2. F3 had a floating lag time of 159 ± 0.12 sec and buoyancy time of 581 ± 0.67 min, in acidic medium and showed no significant changes after 3 months of accelerated stability testing. Hence, the added value of this formulation is the increased retention time of omeprazole in stomach. However, the absence of studies in simulated intestinal fluid leaves some uncertainty about its performance after gastric transit.

Additionally, another study [20] described the formulation of omeprazole magnesium tablets by the solvent evaporation method and direct compression. Six distinct solid dispersion mixtures were prepared, using the excipients ethylcellulose, PVK 314 and MCC, among others, in varying ratios. Post-compression studies about weight variation, content uniformity, thickness, hardness, friability, disintegration, drug content and *in vitro* drug release were conducted. The optimized formulation number 3 (F3), with 15 mg ethylcellulose, was found to have 2% weight variation, 0.25% friability, 21.57 min disintegration time, 99.45% drug content and 98.42% drug release in 6 hours. Although it did not comply with United States Pharmacopeia (USP) standards for hardness, because it was found to have 2.82 kg/cm^3 hardness. Therefore, the added value of this formulation lies in the fact that it presents higher range of drug release capacity at $t = 6$ h, compared to the market formulation, lansoprazole.

At the same time, some studies focused on the use of different/alternative binders and excipients, aiming at enhancing the bioavailability of omeprazole or its release type.

The investigation of Emmanuel et al. [21] on the formulation of omeprazole tablets by direct compression, involved Afzelia gum as a binder, in order to inhibit the gastric degradation of the drug. The main excipients, Afzelia gum and microcrystalline cellulose, were used in different ratios to prepare six different tablet batches. Another batch containing hydroxypropyl methylcellulose, as a binder (Formulation number 7), was also formulated, as control. Fourier-transform infrared spectroscopy indicated the compatibility and stability of the drug within the formulations. The tablets were evaluated for their hardness, friability, porosity, *in vitro* disintegration and *in vitro* drug release. Formulation number 6, with Afzelia gum content of 30%, appears to be suitable to substantially inhibit the gastric degradation of omeprazole. It was found to have 83.4% of drug released and not degraded at $t = 120$ min. On the other hand, it did not pass the tests for crushing strength and friability.

Another study [22] of the same main author describes the formulation of omeprazole tablets using *Prosopis* gum, as a binder, *via* the wet granulation method. Apart from *Prosopis* gum, lactose and magnesium stearate were also included. The granules' flow properties, Hausner's ratio and Carr's index were assessed before compacting them into tables. Then, the physicomechanical properties of the tablets were assessed. Higher concentrations of *Prosopis* gum resulted in greater tensile strength, outperforming hydroxypropyl methylcellulose (HPMC)-based tablets. However, the friability values of all the formulations exceeded the acceptable limit of $\leq$1%. The *in vitro* release profile indicated that formulations with 20% and 30% *Prosopis* gum released 76 and 82% of the drug, respectively, at pH 5.5. Furthermore, the release kinetics studies suggested a diffusion-controlled release mechanism. Thus, the added value of this formulation lies in the alternative excipient, as a means to provide targeted drug delivery.

The study by Bikiaris et al. [23] explored the formulation of chitosan-based omeprazole tablets. Three different tablet formulations were prepared by compression. Each using a distinct type of chitosan (neat, modified with oxidized dextran and modified with oxidized nanocellulose). These formulations also included sodium alginate and lactose monohydrate as excipients. The formulated tablets were evaluated for drug-polymer interactions, crystalline drug structure, swelling behavior, hydrophilicity, cytotoxicity and *in vitro* drug release. Compared to neat chitosan, both derivatives demonstrated low cytotoxicity, notable swelling capacity and increased mucoadhesion. The *in vitro* drug release studies demonstrated erosion, as the primary drug release mechanism and improved dissolution rates at pH 6,8 for the formulations based on the modified chitosan derivatives. Hence, this formulation has the potential for modified-release dosage forms of omeprazole.

Another area of interest was the formulation of tablets through the use of omeprazole-loaded pellets or nanoparticles. The study by Agapakis et al. [24] described six formulations of omeprazole pellet tablets using lactose monohydrate, Avicel® PH-101 and Avicel® PH-102, in varying ratios. All of them were prepared by direct compression, except formulation number 6 (F6), which was prepared by wet granulation. The tablets demonstrated appropriate hardness, uniform size and homogeneity. They were also tested for resistance in pH 4.5 and pH 6.8, and comparisons were made to the brand product Losec®. Formulation F6 had the highest crushing strength and a prolonged release profile, while formulation F7's release rate was comparable to Losec's® (80% within 2 h.). F3 showed a slow, steady release over 4 h, indicating a notable potential in extended-release systems. Intermediate duration release profiles were observed in the remaining formulations. Thermal analyses (thermogravimetric and differential scanning calorimetry) provided insights into the interactions between the excipients and omeprazole, explaining the varying release rates. Overall, the formulated tablets were cost-effective and versatile, making them promising candidates for future applications using other active substances.

The investigation of Parihar et al. [25] explored the formulation of omeprazole magnesium multi-unit particulate tablets. Seal-coated pellets were coated with three layers using the bottom spray technique. Drug layer included HPMC 6cps, IPA and DCM, optimized at 20% HPMC 6cps content (Batch D4). Barrier layer utilized PVA, optimized at 5% content (Batch B7). Enteric coating utilized Eudragit L 100 55, TEX and Plasacrylate T, optimized at 70% weight gain, as it complied with the acid-resistant test (Batch EC3). Then, tablets were prepared by direct compression of 70% enteric-coated pellets with MCC 102, Plasdone K29/32, PEG6000 and sodium stearyl fumarate. Tablet batch number 7 (T7) with a 12% PEG6000 content was found to be optimal, as it released 94.5% of omeprazole in 30 min at pH 6.8. Electron microscopy showed that the pellets maintained their spherical morphology during the compression, while Fourier-transform infrared spectroscopy and differential scanning calorimetry confirmed no drug-excipient interaction. Furthermore, T7 showed no significant changes after 1 month of accelerated stability testing. Therefore, this formulation offers a multi-unit particulate system approach for enhanced controlled release.

The study by Juère et al. [26] examined the formulation of tablets consisting of omeprazole-loaded mesoporous silica nanoparticles (dendritic and MCM-48-type) combined with succinylated β-lactoglobulin (BL).

First the two types of MSNs were synthesized and then both were additionally functionalized with HMDS. Rotary evaporation led to the encapsulation of omeprazole into the MSNs. Then, drug-loaded MSNs and BL powders were physically mixed together and compressed directly into tablets. *In vitro* drug release studies showed that the DMSN-based tablet met the United States Pharmacopeia (USP) standards for gastroresistance, while at pH 7.4, the formulation led to the release of omeprazole (76%) over 8 hours, with functionalization affecting release rates; methylated DMSNs show lower release (55 vs. 76%). In the cytotoxicity studies, it was found that pure MSNs are non-cytotoxic but the functionalization enhanced cytotoxicity. Thus, the formulation provides improved drug stability in the gastric environment. Furthermore, the functionalized MSNs could be used in applications, where higher cell mortality is desirable.

Similarly, another study [27] investigated the formulation of omeprazole-loaded silver nanoparticle tablets using gelatin and sodium alginate, as enteric coating polymers. Five distinct powder formulations were prepared into tablets. However, the specific ratios of the excipients used were not provided. Post-compression studies indicated that all batches met the acceptable criteria. In the *in vitro* drug release studies, batch formulation number 4, which contained 4% sodium alginate and 5% gelatin, demonstrated optimal performance with negligible drug release in 0.1 N HCl and 98% release in phosphate buffer, over a 12-hour period. In consequence, the added value of this formulation lies on its use of natural polymers in advanced drug delivery systems, showcasing significant controlled release of the drug.

Innovative approaches were also made in the area of capsule formulations, in order to improve the drug's release and bioavailability. The study by Chandra et al. [28] detailed the formulation of omeprazole microballon-loaded capsules using the emulsion solvent diffusion method. Six distinct microballoon formulations were created by using varying ratios of ethyl cellulose and HPMC K4M, which were the main excipients used. The resultant microballoon powders were encapsulated in capsule shells. Fourier-transform infrared spectroscopy confirmed compatibility between omeprazole and the excipients. Various preformulation parameters including the micromeritic properties, particle size, entrapment efficiency, SEM, yield percentage and *in vitro* buoyancy were assessed. Formulation number 6-F6 (4:1 ratio of ethyl cellulose to HPMC4) was optimized due to its appropriate characteristics and demonstration of a maximum release of 90.19 ± 0.48% in 6 h, at pH 1.2. Drug release kinetics indicated the highest regression coefficient values for the first-order model, suggesting diffusion as the primary drug release mechanism. Thus, this formulation presents enhanced bioavailability *via* prolonged gastric residence time.

Another investigation [29] examined the formulation of a delayed-release omeprazole dosage form using ready-to-fill functional EUDRACAP® enteric capsules, which are pre-locked HPMC capsules with the Eudragit polymer coating and provide up to 4 hours of acid resistance, precise pH-targeted release and easy manual filling without the need for banding. Their acid resistance was tested in a 0.1 N HCl medium for over 2 hours, showing less than 10% drug release, meeting the criteria for acidic conditions. Furthermore, impurity levels after exposure to acidic stress were at 0.22%, well within the 2.00% limit, demonstrating excellent protection by EUDRACAP®. Comparative analysis of the *in vitro* performance indicated higher acid protection over commercial products. In conclusion, the added value of this formulation lies on its viability as an alternative for enteric dosage forms, suitable for both large-scale and small-pharmacy productions.

Similarly, the study by Kumisbek et al. [30] investigated the formulation of a bioequivalent delayed-release omeprazole capsule filled with omeprazole pellets. Microcrystalline cellulose pellets were coated using the fluidized bed method with three distinct layers: active (omeprazole), protective (hydroxypropylmethylcellulose) and enteric (Eudragit L30-D55, PlasAcryl, Titanium dioxide). Comparative studies were performed on the generic formulation (40 mg) *versus* Losec® (40 mg, two

20 mg capsules). Dissolution studies at pH 1.2 showed 1.3–5.7% omeprazole release after 120 minutes, while at pH 6.8, 90.8–92.3% was released, with >85% released within 15 minutes. Stability studies, including dissolution, acid resistance, buffer stage, impurity assay and microbiological purity tests, confirmed compliance with all specifications over 6-month accelerated and 12-month long-term studies. Packaging used high-density polyethylene bottles and aluminum foil blisters. A bioequivalence study with 24 healthy volunteers, using a crossover design, confirmed the bioequivalence of the generic, with a 24-month shelf life.

Other investigations have also focused on the size of the capsule, like the study by Geng et al. [31], which describes the formulation of a lightweight omeprazole capsule. To enhance its solubility and stability, omeprazole was encapsulated in β-cyclodextrin (β-CD). The effect of molar ratios of omeprazole and β-CD, inclusion time and temperature on the efficiency of encapsulation was assessed. Optimal conditions were found to be: stirring omeprazole and β-CD at a 1:2 molar ratio at 30°C for 3 hours. Fourier-transform infrared spectroscopy, differential scanning calorimetry and X-ray diffraction were used to evaluate omeprazole inclusions. Furthermore, based on the pH-time curves magnesium oxide and sodium bicarbonate were chosen among other anti-acid materials to reduce the weight of the capsule contents. *In vitro* drug release studies revealed significantly improved drug dissolution and bioavailability, with a release rate of 95.42 ± 2.51% in a simulated gastric environment. *In vivo* pharmacokinetics in rabbits showed a significant increase in AUC0-t compared to the market capsule (ENCHENG®). In conclusion, this lightweight formulation presents a promising oral delivery system.

In another advanced approach [32], omeprazole loaded with gum Arabic (GA)—*O*-carboxymethyl chitosan (OCMC) microcapsules, was used. The methods involved a layer-by-layer (LbL) assembly and genipin crosslinking. SPAN60 and soybean oil were the rest excipients. CLSM verified that the LbL microcapsules were effectively created, displaying a core-shell structure. Furthermore, studies about the microcapsules' properties and their *in vitro* swelling behavior revealed no influence of genipin crosslinking on their encapsulation efficiency or drug loading but a decreased particle size and positive charge. Crosslinking also enhanced their stability in simulated gastric fluid. An increased bioavailability of omeprazole was demonstrated by the pharmacokinetic studies in mice, with 0,1 mg/mL genipin crosslinking yielding the highest relative to the control formulation bioavailability of 8,76. The added value of this formulation lies in its potential for oral delivery of nutraceuticals. It also has an adjustable delivery performance *via* varying genipin crosslinking degree.

Lastly, the investigation of Sanni et al. [33] describes the formulation of a combined dosage form (caplet), comprising diclofenac sodium mini tablet and omeprazole sodium pellets loaded in capsule shells. Wet granulation method was used to prepare the mini tablet of diclofenac sodium using HPMC, PVP K30 and MCC in varying ratios, creating nine distinct formulations. Through extensive evaluation, all batches met pharmacopeia standards for thickness, weight variation, hardness, friability, drug content and *in vitro* drug release. The optimized formulation, F3 (HPMC: PVP: MCC = 24: 16: 57 mg), exhibited a maximum diclofenac release of 97,84% over 12 hours. Enteric-coated omeprazole pellets were directly purchased from a wholesale trader and, alongside one diclofenac sodium tablet, were encapsulated in size 0 capsule shells. The *in vitro* drug release studies of the pallets revealed the maximum omeprazole release to be 1,17% in acidic medium within 2 h and 93,07% within 1 h in buffer medium. Therefore, the formulation presents to minimize the gastric side effects of diclofenac sodium and decrease its frequency of administration.

In conclusion, regarding solid formulations, there is another noteworthy study by Kim et al. [34], which describes the formulation of an oral thin film composed of omeprazole and seaweed calcium (SC). First, the SC was obtained from lyophilized seaweed *via* ultra-multiple crystal method. Then, a solid dispersion of omeprazole and SC was prepared and mixed with mannitol, crospovidone, kollidon SR, MgSt and PEG. Various polymers, such as Kollidon® VA64, PVP K-30, HPMC 4 K and HPMC 100 K, were then added as binders to form four different batches (BAT1–4). Then, the other thin films were fabricated using a heating press and deep freezing. Dissolution testing and high-performance liquid chromatography confirmed drug efficiency in all batches. However, BAT 3 was found to be the optimal formulation, having the highest dissolution rate and suitable properties in XRD, TGA, DSC and FTIR analyses. This formulation offers rapid dissolution and absorption in the oral cavity and has potential to mitigate the calcium deficiency side effects of omeprazole therapy.

2.2.2 Semi-solid formulations

In the field of semi-solid formulation have been significant innovative approaches, both in enhancing omeprazole bioavailability and delivery, as well as in repurposing it.

The study by Rouaz-El Hajoui et al. [35] explores and compares the formulation of two semi-solid omeprazole formulations: chewable hydrogels (Formulation 1/F1) and chewable enteric pellets (Formulation 2/F2) using 3D printing technology. For F1 the process began with a three-layer coating (drug layer, protective layer and enteric layer) of microcrystalline cellulose pellets *via* bottom spray coating technique, using hypromellose, sodium citrate and Eudragit® L-30 D-55. Next, pharmaceutical inks were prepared for both formulations using carrageenan and xanthan gum. Additionally, F1 included carboxymethyl cellulose, sodium bicarbonate and glycerol, while F2 incorporated gelatin and lemon juice. Both formulations exhibited appropriate rheology and printability, and met content and mass uniformity standards, but F1 was found to melt quickly with body warmth (>5 min holding). Dissolution, drug release and gastroresistance were examined, revealing that F1 was not gastro-resistant. Conversely, the high gastroresistance and suitable release profile of F2 make it a viable candidate for addressing pediatric medication challenges, as it can be administered at variable doses, and has eye-catching appearance and good organoleptic properties.

Another investigation [36] details the formulation of an omeprazole magnesium *in situ* gel. Nine formulations were made with varying concentrations of sodium alginate, tri-sodium citrate, calcium carbonate and water. Fourier-transform infrared spectroscopy confirmed no interaction between the excipients and omeprazole. Formulation F6 (sodium alginate: calcium carbonate, 2:1) was selected as optimal due to its highest *in vitro* drug release and favorable physicochemical properties such as color, pH, homogeneity, floating lag time, floating duration and drug content. Furthermore, a comparative study on drug content and *in vitro* drug release and kinetic modeling between F6 and a marketed formulation was conducted, suggesting that the *in situ* gel formulation is a viable alternative, offering desirable physicochemical properties, high bioavailability and sustained drug release.

Additionally, the study by Heikal et al. [37] explores the formulation of chitosan-coated hydrogel beads loaded with omeprazole (OMP) and curcumin (CURC), aiming to enhance the anti-ulcerogenic impact of these compounds. Initially, OMP and CURC were complexed with hydroxypropyl-β-cyclodextrin. Then, the complex was loaded into alginate beads and coated with chitosan and CaCl2 solution. Fourier-transform infrared spectroscopy confirmed no incompatibility between excipients and active pharmaceutical ingredients. The optimal formulation (F8) (sodium alginate 3%, CaCl2 4%, CS 0,5%), which was selected *via* Design-Expert® software, showed an encapsulation efficiency of approx. 87,44%, swelling of approx. 800%, and a diameter of 2,60 mm. In the *in vitro* drug release studies F8 showed a release of 23,19% for CURC and 17,19% for OMP after 2 h, and 87,81% for CURC and 81,67% for OMP after 24 h. *In vitro* bioadhesion test, *in vivo* treatment efficacy study and histological examination confirmed bioadhesive characteristics, and higher antiulcer effectiveness of F8 compared to free OMP, CURC-only beads and OMP-only beads. Therefore, the added value of this formulation lies in its potential as an alternative for managing peptic ulcers.

Furthermore, another study [38] examines the formulation of a tamarind seed gum-based omeprazole magnesium-loaded hydrogel. Eight distinct hydrogel formulations were synthesized using varying concentrations of Tamarind seed gum (TG) 2-Acrylamido-2-methyl propane sulfonic acid (AMPS), N,N-methylene bis acrylamide (MBA) and ammonium persulfate (APS) *via* free radical graft copolymerization of AMPS onto the TG backbone. F4 formulation with TG:AMPS:MBA:APS ratio to be 0,15: 0,35: 0,02: 0,01 was found to have optimum swelling at pH 7, drug loading 70 ± 1% within 48 h and drug release 97,85 ± 1% over 1200 min at pH 1,5, adhering to the Hill equation model. *In vivo* toxicity tests using a Drosophila model confirmed no toxicity at tested concentrations. These findings demonstrate the potential of this formulation for controlled and targeted drug delivery applications.

On the other hand, focusing on repurposing, the study by Ullah et al. [39] describes the formulation of a chitosan-coated omeprazole-loaded nanoemulgel for skin and soft tissue infections. Initially, three distinct omeprazole nanoemulsion formulations were prepared *via* high-pressure/speed homogenization, comprising chitosan and olive oil in varying concentrations. The optimal formulation (OMP3NE) had a ratio of 10:15:3,5:71,2 w/w of Olive Oil:Tween 80:Span 80:distilled water. The nanoemulgel (OMP3NEG) was then prepared by mixing OMP3NE with a Carbopol® gelling solution, stirring and adding triethanolamine. Fourier-transform infrared spectroscopy confirmed no incompatibility between excipients and omeprazole. OMP3NEG was then characterized for zeta potential, size distribution, pH, drug content, entrapment efficiency, viscosity, spreadability and extrudability, all within acceptable ranges. *In vitro* drug release study showed 82,16% at pH 5,5 after 24 hours. The microbiological assay showed that MIC results (1,25 mg/mL) against *Escherichia coli* (Gram-negative bacterium involved in both symbiotic and pathogenic interactions within humans), *Klebsiella pneumoniae* (Gram-negative bacterium often associated with hospital-acquired infections), *Pseudomonas aeruginosa* (Gram-negative bacterium known for its biofilm formation and intrinsic resistance to antibiotics) and *Staphylococcus aureus* (Gram-positive bacterium responsible for various infections ranging from superficial skin infections to severe systemic diseases) were satisfactory, and also chitosan coating enhanced omeprazole's antibacterial activity.

Hence, the added value of this formulation lies in its potent repurposing of omeprazole for topical delivery.

Additionally, another study [40] explores the formulation of injectable omeprazole-loaded hydrogels for potential pancreatitis treatment. The excipients used include hyaluronic acid (HA), H2L, β-diketone (acetylacetone) and carbonyl dihydrazine (CDH). Applying H2L and β-diketone together formed a coordinator complex, followed by a crosslinking reaction between oxidized HA (OHA) and CDH-HA, creating the injectable HA hydrogel. The exact stage at which omeprazole is loaded is not specified in the text. SEM analysis revealed the hydrogel's three-dimensional network internal microstructure and macroporous architecture. Cell Counting Kit-8 (CCK-8) and Elisa assays were performed to assess the hydrogel's biological activity on pancreatitis cells compared to the control. CCK-8 showed higher cell viability, which increased alongside hydrogel concentration. Experiments with Elisa® confirmed a significant reduction in inflammatory cytokine release. These findings suggest the formulation as a promising candidate for treating pancreatitis.

Furthermore, the study by Kathiravan [41] details the formulation of a combined omeprazole/acyclovir nanogel by solvent diffusion method for transdermal delivery. Nine distinct formulations were prepared using Carbopol® 940, tragacanth gum, propylene glycol and triethanolamine in different ratios. Fourier-transform infrared spectroscopy showed no incompatibility between active pharmaceutical ingredients and excipients. Many other studies have been conducted, assessing pH, homogeneity, spreadability, viscosity, percentage yield and drug content. The optimized formulation number 9 (F9) (with a ratio of 100:100:1:1 Carbopol ®940:tragacanth gum: propylene glycol: triethanolamine) with pH 6,9 and drug content of 92,65% exhibited the best release rates with a sustained release profile, achieving 99% for acyclovir and 97,5% for omeprazole at the end of 24 hours outperforming a marketed formulation (acyclovir alone), which could lead to increased antiviral activity.

Moving to other semi-solid formulations, there is the formulation of omeprazole buccal foams, as described in the study by Chachlioutaki et al. [42]. Five foams were created from lyophilized aqueous gels of maltodextrin with HPMC, L-arginine, sodium lauryl sulfate, sodium taurocholate and croscarmellose, with four also containing either sodium alginate, chitosan, porcine gelatin or tragacanth gum. Studies conducted included X-ray diffraction, Fourier-transform infrared spectroscopy, differential scanning calorimetry, rheological, mucoadhesion, *in vitro* dissolution and disintegration, high-performance liquid chromatography and *ex vivo* permeability tests. The HPMC-Alg-OME foam was identified as optimal, meeting effective buccal drug delivery criteria with moderate hardness, high porosity and strong mucoadhesion, leading to prolonged residence time and enhanced drug transport across the epithelium. It also increased the drug's apparent permeability by 30 times compared to the drug suspension. Additionally, all foams exhibited excellent stability, with omeprazole content unchanged after 6 months at 20°C and 45% RH. Thus, this formulation has the potential to address stability and administration issues, particularly benefiting children and the elderly with swallowing difficulties.

Lastly, another investigation [43] examines the formulation of an omeprazole suppository for infants with gastroesophageal reflux disease (GERD).

The excipients used were Witepsol H15 and L-arginine base, with the optimal formulation achieved by pouring at 34.7°C and stirring at 200 rpm. The suppositories displayed excellent stability, with no discoloration and unchanged omeprazole content after 1 year stored in the dark at room temperature. Effectiveness and pharmacokinetic data were provided in an accompanying article by the same authors, "Rectal Omeprazole in Infants With gastroesophageal reflux disease: A Randomized Pilot Trial," published in the European Journal of Drug Metabolism and Pharmacokinetics (2020), showing that a 1 mg/kg dose results in rapid therapeutic exposure. In conclusion, this formulation presents a promising alternative for infants with severe GERD.

2.3 Nanoformulations

This chapter overviews various nanoformulations of omeprazole made in the last 5 years, including nanoparticles, nanobullets and liposomes. Collectively, these formulations represent significant advancements in pharmaceutical technology, approaching key challenges in drug delivery and efficacy. Some of them also focus on the innovative field of drug repurposing.

To begin with, the study by Khatibi et al. [44] presents the formulation of omeprazole-loaded cellulose acetate phthalate nanoparticles (CAP NPs) using microfluidic (MF) and bulk (BM) nanoprecipitation methods. Characterization revealed that MF produced more uniform and smaller particles (average diameter of 65 ± 6 nm) with higher encapsulation efficiency (EE of 68,26 ± 2,03%) and loading capacity (LC of 11,34 ± 0.96%) compared to BM. Fourier-transform infrared spectroscopy confirmed no interaction between omeprazole and the polymer in MF OME-CAP NPs. *In vitro* release studies showed that MF OME-CAP NPs released 9,24% of omeprazole at pH 1,2 and 85.66% at pH 7,4, compared to 18,89 and 95,18% for BM OME-CAP NPs. *In vivo* antiulcer evaluations revealed that MF OME-CAP NPs had an ulcer index of 10,26 and the highest protection rate of 82,26%, with minimal gastric damage in histological studies. Thus, the MF method provided controlled release and superior antiulcer activity compared to BM and free omeprazole, making MF OME-CAP NPs a promising nanocarrier for antiulcer therapy.

Another study [45] describes the formulation of enteric-coated omeprazole-loaded nanoparticles using Eudragit L 100–55 (EU) and chitosan *via* a complex coacervation method. A three-level factorial design evaluated the impact of EU concentration and EU/CTS ratio on OMP-NPs' properties. Characterization showed particle sizes ranging from 618 nm to 996 nm, increasing with higher EU concentrations and ratios. Zeta potential values also increased with higher EU levels, indicating improved stability. Entrapment efficiency ranged from 55–93%, and drug loading varied from 5,5 to 18,9%. Dissolution studies revealed approximately 70% omeprazole release at pH 6,8 over 24 hours.

Optimization identified the F5 formulation (EU 4 mg/mL, EU/CTS ratio 2:1) as optimal, with a desirability factor of 0,85 and minimal errors in PS (2,65%), ZP (15,7%), EE% (12,3%) and DL% (15,4%). SEM analysis showed spherical nanoparticles under 300 nm. *In vivo* studies confirmed that OMP-NPs significantly reduced ulcer area and severity, improved histopathological scores and increased gastric pH (7,2 ± 1,3 for nanoparticles, 6,8 ± 0,9 for pellets and 2,1 ± 0,1 for controls). These findings suggest optimized nanoparticles could effectively treat ulcers.

Additionally, the investigation by Li et al. [46] explores the formulation of omeprazole (OME)—*Bletilla striata* polysaccharide (BSP) nanoparticles by inverse emulsion and surface crosslinking methods. The main excipients used were BSP, carboxymethyl chitosan, sodium alginate and Span-80. *In vitro* stability studies showed that the OME-BSP NPs reduced OME degradation by 22% at 2 hours in acidic conditions and allowed sustained release for up to 24 hours. *In situ* gastric absorption study in ethanol-induced gastric ulcered rats showed that they increased OME absorption by 2,6 times (42,57%) compared to free OME. Pharmacokinetic studies revealed a twofold increase in AUC and a threefold extended half-life. Moreover, the formulated nanoparticles effectively inhibited H^+-K^+ -ATPase activity, raising gastric pH and improving acid suppression. They significantly reduced gastric ulcer scores from 4,25 to 1,17, as confirmed by histopathological analysis. Additional studies demonstrated reduced cell apoptosis and enhanced antioxidant and anti-inflammatory responses, highlighting their potential for targeted gastric ulcer treatment.

Furthermore, another study [47] details the formulation of chitosan nanoparticles (CSNPS) loaded with omeprazole (OME) and ammonium tetrathiomolybdate (ATM) for gastric ulcer treatment. The formulation was achieved *via* ionic gelation with tripolyphosphate (TPP) as a crosslinker. Then the nanoparticles were characterized by UV-visible (UV–vis) spectroscopy, FTIR, XRD and HPLC, confirming successful crosslinking and drug encapsulation (OME EE 65,3 ± 2,25% and ATM adsorption 74,33 ± 3,38%). The release of ATM was sustained, with 25,8% released over 72 hours. MTT assay showed that CSNPS-OME-ATM nanoparticles had a higher IC50 than ATM alone, indicating enhanced cytoprotective effects. *In vivo* studies with indomethacin-induced gastric ulcers in rats revealed significant reduction in ulcerative lesions and improved histopathological outcomes with CSNPS-OME-ATM, demonstrating its potential for effective gastric ulcer treatment.

Moreover, the study by Moretto et al. [48] describes the formulation of omeprazole-loaded supermagnetic multi-core-shell nanoparticles (MMCSNPs) for controlled drug delivery. MMCSNPs were synthesized through a five-step process: sol-gel synthesis of NiFe cores, silica and phenolic resin coating, carbonization, silica etching and surface functionalization (Pluronic® F-127). Characterization confirmed the success of each preparation step. TEM verified the multi-core structure and consistent particle size (diameter of 25,09 nm). Fourier-transform infrared spectroscopy confirmed the silica removal and successful functionalization. Thermogravimetric analysis (TGA) indicated successful carbonization. Additionally, magnetic characterization revealed a saturation magnetization of ~43 $A{\cdot}m^2/kg$, ensuring effective magnetic drug targeting (MDT). Drug loading efficiency was 51,35%, with a maximum cumulative release of 61,5% at pH = 7,4 over 48 hours, following the Fickian diffusion mechanism. Thus, the formulated nanoparticles show potential for targeted drug delivery.

Building on this, the following studies have explored different nanoformulation strategies, aiming to investigate omeprazole repurposing and therapeutic potential.

The study by Sun et al. [49] details the formulation of omeprazole liposomes *via* thin film hydration method to explore a novel drug delivery platform for acute lung injury (ALI). The liposomes, incorporating cholesterol and phosphatidylcholine, resulted in Nano-omeprazole (Nano-OM), which effectively targeted lung macrophages and exhibited significant anti-inflammatory activity by inhibiting Toll-like receptor (TLR) signaling pathways. *In vitro* assays, confirmed by flow cytometry and confocal microscopy, demonstrated Nano-OM uptake by lung macrophages. Cytokine analysis in an ALI mouse model showed that Nano-OM significantly reduced inflammatory markers, such as TNF-α and IL-6, in bronchoalveolar lavage fluid (BALF). Histopathological analysis further confirmed reduced lung tissue damage. Thus, these findings suggest that through drug repurposing Nano-OM is a promising therapeutic strategy for ALI.

Furthermore, the study by Eswar et al. [50] describes the formulation of omeprazole-loaded cooper nanoparticles by thin film hydration method. It also evaluates their synergistic anticancer activity. Firstly, the cooper nanoparticles were modified with L-cysteine (CCuNPs). Then, HSPC, CCuNPs and omeprazole were used in a ratio of 10:1:2 to create the thin film. Various studies were conducted to evaluate the synergistic anticancer activity of omeprazole and CCuNPs against B16 melanoma cells, such as MTT Assay, Live/Dead Assay, DCHFDA Assay, JC-1 Assay, AO/EtBr Staining, Flow Cytometry Analysis and Clonogenic Assay. The results of the above-mentioned studies suggest that this nanosystem is highly promising as a single platform to deliver two active pharmaceutical ingredients, exhibiting synergistic activity for substantial damage to the mitochondria of the cancer cells (enhanced reactive oxygen species (ROS) generation) and induction of necrotic cell death. Consequently, this formulation has potential for further investigation as an anticancer agent.

Additionally, another investigation [51] details the formulation of human serum albumin (HSA)-coated, omeprazole (OME)-loaded tellurium double-headed nanobullets (TeDNBs) and explores their tumor therapeutic potential. TeDNBs are synthesized by reacting tellurium dioxide, selenous acid and hydrazine hydrate (80%), followed by termination with sodium lauryl sulfate and purification. TeDNBs-HO are then prepared by dispersing TeDNBs in water, incorporating HSA, mixing with omeprazole and purifying. UV-vis spectra demonstrated effective, time- and concentration-dependent hydrogen peroxide (H_2O_2) depletion by TeDNBs. Morphological and structural analyses *via* transmission electron microscopy (TEM), scanning electron microscopy (SEM), and X-ray diffraction analysis (XRD) were complemented by X-ray photoelectron spectroscopy (XPS), which confirmed Te(IV) oxidation after H_2O_2 reaction. TeDNBs exhibited significant H_2O_2 degradation, glutathione (GSH) depletion, photothermal conversion efficiency of 29,71%, and a drug loading capacity of 29.608%. Near-infrared (NIR) irradiation notably enhanced OME release nearly twice. Endocytosis studies showed TeDNBs-HO accumulation in lysosomes. High cytotoxicity was observed in 4 T1 cells (36,65% viability) under near-infrared region spectroscopy (NIR), while human umbilical vein endothelial cells (HUVECs) showed minimal toxicity (82,12% viability). TeDNBs-HO induced endoplasmic reticulum stress, autophagy dysfunction and lysosomal impairment. *In vivo* imaging (CT, MSOT) indicated peak signals at 6 hours, with inductively coupled plasma mass spectrometry (ICP-MS) revealing 20,78% ID/g Te in tumors. Thus, TeDNBs-HO have potency as theranostics and tumor-therapeutics.

Moreover, the study by Sharifzadeh et al. [52] describes the formulation of silver nanoparticles (AgNPs) functionalized with omeprazole (Ag@Omp) and omeprazole sulfide (Ag@Omps). The synthesis involved reducing AgNO3 with NaBH4 in the presence of polyvinylpyrrolidone, followed by drug incorporation. X-ray diffraction confirmed the nanoparticles' face-centered cubic structure. UV-vis absorption spectra and TEM imaging confirmed the formation of Ag-drug complexes, with spherical particles sized <40 nm for Ag@Omp and < 60 nm for Ag@Omps. Antibacterial studies conducted showed that AgNPs significantly enhanced the antibacterial properties of both drugs, with Ag@Omps demonstrating superior activity. Therefore, these formulations show potential as antibacterial agents.

Expanding on this concept, another study of the same authors [53] describes the formulation of silver nanoparticles (SNPs) using leaf extracts from different plants: Ruta, mango and Pimpinella saxifrage, functionalized with omeprazole and omeprazole sulfide. The SNPs were synthesized by mixing plant extracts with a silver nitrate solution, followed by drug incorporation. Although their exact size and shape were not specified, the presence of distinct surface plasmon resonance (SPR) peaks and functional group interactions confirmed their successful synthesis and stability. UV-vis spectra confirmed the reduction of silver nitrate, while Fourier-transform infrared spectroscopy revealed characteristic signals indicating successful silver-drug attachment. In conclusion, the study highlights the potential of plant-mediated synthesis for creating eco-friendly, drug-loaded SNPs with enhanced therapeutic properties (antibacterial properties, as mentioned above).

Similarly, the study by Zia et al. [54] explores also the formulation of omeprazole-loaded silver nanoparticles (Omp-AgNPs). The Omp-AgNPs were synthesized by mixing $AgNO_3$ and omeprazole solutions (1:3 ratio), followed by reduction using $NaBH_4$, confirmed by a UV-vis spectrum peak at 421 nm. Omp-AgNPs were found to be stable at pH 6–7, but unstable at pH 2–3 and pH 12–13, high temperatures, and at all concentrations of NaCl solution (0,5 to 2 M). Fourier-transform infrared spectroscopy (FTIR), X-ray diffraction analysis (XRD) and transmission electron microscopy (TEM) analyses revealed key functional groups involved in stabilization, a cubic crystalline structure and spherical particles averaging 17 nm in size. Omp-AgNPs exhibited 80,23% urease inhibition and 84,45% radical scavenging activity, compared to 69,45% and 72,21% for omeprazole alone. Antibacterial tests showed inhibition zones of 13,6 mm (*E. coli*) and 12 mm (*S. aureus*). These results suggest that Omp-AgNPs have potential as antibacterial, antioxidant and urease inhibitory agents.

2.4 Liquid formulations

This chapter overviews various liquid formulations of omeprazole made in the last 5 years. All of them being liquid inherently offer administration flexibility and some of them utilize also pellets and nanoparticles.

To begin with, the study by Mobarak Qamsari et al. [55] describes the formulation of a *Lactobacillus acidophilus* ATCC 4356 surface layer protein coated omeprazole suspension. Initially, the omeprazole powder was analyzed for melting point, infrared (IR) and ultraviolet (UV) spectra and particle size, followed by size reduction, achieving an optimal 35,516 μm average particle size. The one-variable-at-a-time method was used to assess the impact of various factors on the coating process, including the type of coating method, amount of S-layer protein, time, temperature, shaking rate, different concentrations of EDTA and sodium taurocholate and the effect of various sugars as binding agents. Furthermore, the stability of the coated omeprazole was tested at pH 5. Optimal coating conditions involved using extracted from the dialysis process S-layer protein monomers at a 2:1 ratio to omeprazole for 2 hours at 25°C, with a shaking rate of 100 rpm in a 50 mM Tris hydrochloride buffer at pH 8. EDTA concentrations did not affect the efficiency, while sodium taurocholate initially protected the drug but eventually had a destructive effect. Sugars also did not improve the coating process. The coating reduced omeprazole's decomposition rate by up to 2223 times and therefore has potential to increase the stability of other unstable drugs.

Additionally, the investigation of Ronchi et al. [56] explores the formulation of an omeprazole-based liquid oral dosage form designed for delayed release. The process utilizes fluid bed-coated, multi-layered particles suspended in syrup. Uniform-sized microcrystalline cellulose pellets were chosen as the core. A first layer containing omeprazole, PVP and talc was applied. To prevent light degradation, a second layer of PVP, talc and titanium dioxide was added. For gastroresistance, a third layer of Eudragit® L100-55, ATEC and talc ensured delayed release at pH 6,8. A fourth layer of PVP and talc prevented interaction between the third and fifth layers. The fifth layer, with Eudragit® E100 and talc, prevented premature omeprazole release in syrup and its degradation in acidic environment. The particles were then suspended in a syrup base of Neosorb sorbitol, Avicel® RC-591, Kollidon® K30, anhydrous sodium and carbonate disodium. The process achieved a 90% yield and particle size below 500 μm, with stability for 10 days at ambient temperature. Stability tests confirmed the protection of the active pharmaceutical ingredient in acidic conditions and effective intestinal release, offering a patient-friendly solution for those with swallowing difficulties.

Another study utilizing pellets [57] describes the formulation of two liquid omeprazole oral solutions (Formulations A and B) for pediatric use. Formulation A used crushed omeprazole pellets, while Formulation B employed pure omeprazole. Both contained mainly sorbitol, glycerin, sodium carboxymethyl cellulose and sodium saccharin, among other excipients. Stored at 4°C and 25°C, omeprazole content was assessed *via* micro-high-performance liquid chromatography at intervals up to 150 days. Formulation A remained stable for 150 days at 4°C and 14 days at 25°C, while Formulation B remained stable for 90 days at 4°C but only 1 day at 25°C. Various parameters, including appearance, flavor, pH, viscosity and resuspendibility, were evaluated. Additionally, microbiological studies were performed per United States Pharmacopeia (USP) guidelines. Formulation A at both temperatures and Formulation B at 4°C met the specifications for microbial examination of non-sterile products over 150 days. In conclusion, both formulations are suitable for pediatric patients, with Formulation A offering superior room temperature stability and preferable taste.

Moreover, the study by Denga et al. [58] investigates the formulation of omeprazole niosome solution using the thin film method to enhance its delivery. The process involves optimizing the ratio of Tween-80 to cholesterol (3:1) and refining hydration conditions, achieving a high encapsulation efficiency of 92,40% for omeprazole vesicles. The vesicles are produced with an average diameter of 70 nm. Comprehensive characterization through TEM, IR and TG confirms successful encapsulation and the structural integrity of the vesicles. *In vitro* release studies at pH 6.8 showed that omeprazole vesicles had an enhanced release time (75 min), release rate (33,19%) and sudden release phenomenon compared to pure omeprazole. Therefore, the formulated system presents to improve omeprazole's release characteristics.

In the study by Gupta et al. [59], the formulation of an omeprazole-loaded nanosuspension is described. Twelve formulations were prepared using Poloxamer 407, HPMC K100M or PVA in different ratios *via* precipitation ultrasonication method. The formulation number 10/F10 (omeprazole to PVA ratio 1:2, had a particle size of 198.6 nm, entrapment efficiency of 88,9% and *in vitro* drug release of 82,2% at 60 min) was found to be optimal. Statistical optimization using a 2^2 factorial design identified the best conditions as 90 mg PVA and 40 minutes of sonication. Regression analysis showed that the particles had a size of 175 nm and a zeta potential of −24.5 mV. The *in vitro* drug release rate was 87,3% and the entrapment efficiency was 92,7%, indicating that R2 formulation was the most effective. No significant changes were indicated by the stability studies about the controlled drug release pattern or entrapment efficiency over a 3-month period. Consequently, the formulation is suitable for large-scale manufacturing and can be adapted for injectable nanosuspensions since PVA is suitable for parenteral administration.

Similarly, the study by Diefenthaeler et al. [60] describes the formulation of enteric-coated omeprazole nanoparticles *via* the nanoprecipitation method for a pediatric-friendly liquid dosage form. Excipients included Eudragit® RS100 (inner core), Eudragit® L100-55 (outer coat), polysorbate 80, sodium bicarbonate and peanut oil. The formulated nanoparticles had a spherical morphology (Transmission electron microscopy/TEM confirmed), mean diameter of 174 ± 17 nm, zeta potential of −13 ± 2,60 mV and 68,1% encapsulation efficiency (when EL100-55 was 0,03%). Stability tests showed no significant changes over 60 days. *In vitro* release studies showed less than 11% drug release at pH 1,2 but significant release (73 ± 3,1%) at pH 6,8 within 60 minutes, indicating also a sustained release profile. Brine shrimp lethality assay showed less than 10% mortality, indicating no toxicity. *In vivo* toxicity assay in mice showed no clinical signs of toxicity, normal body weight and hematologic parameters. *In vivo* antiulcer activity studies showed that nanoparticles significantly reduced ethanol-induced gastric ulcer areas, with a protection percentage of 93,08%, higher than omeprazole alone (29,71%).

In conclusion, these findings suggest a promising formulation for pediatric administration.

Lastly, an innovative approach [61] investigated the formulation of an omeprazole-based radio solution for targeting and imaging peptic ulcers. A [99mTc] tricarbonyl core was used to prepare [^{99m}Tc]tricarbonyl omeprazole complex.

Thin layer chromatography (TLC) and high-performance liquid chromatography confirmed a 98,0% radiochemical conversion and also assessed the complex's stability in rat serum media, showing 96% radiochemical purity for up to 24 hours, decreasing to 88,0% at 48 hours.

Furthermore, biodistribution studies were conducted on Swiss Albino mice, including normal, chemically ulcerated (ethanol) and microbially ulcerated (*H. pylori*) groups. Stomach uptake for each group was found to be 10,5, 29,6 and 38,7% ID/g at 1 h after intravenous injection, respectively. Thus, the added value of this formulation lies in its potential as a highly selective peptic ulcer radiotracer, particularly in microbially ulcerated group.

2.5 Other formulations

In this chapter, there is an overview of other omeprazole formulations made in the last 5 years, including pellets, microsphere, salts and co-crystals.

2.5.1 Pellet formulations

First the study by Anusha et al. [62] details the formulation of sustained-release omeprazole pellets using the extrusion and spheronization method. Nine distinct formulations were created using sodium bicarbonate, microcrystalline cellulose (MCC), talc and starch and one of the following polymers in varying ratios: HPMC K15M, HPMC K100 or HPMC E15. Fourier-transform infrared spectroscopy and differential scanning calorimetry studies confirmed no interaction between the drug and the excipients. The formulated pellets were assessed for their loose and tapped bulk density, compressibility index, angle of repose, friability, drug content, moisture content and loss on drying. Furthermore, *in vitro* drug release studies were conducted in 0,1 N HCl for 12 hours. The optimized formulation, F1 (HPMC K15M = 25 mg), produced pellets with acceptable characteristics, drug content, low friability, and it was found to follow zero-order kinetics.

F1 demonstrated an 89,14% drug release at 12 hours, which was more sustained compared to the innovator (89,8% drug release at 8 hours). Thus, the formulation has potential to outperform the conventional dosage form.

Additionally, another study [63] describes the formulation of enteric polymer-coated omeprazole pellets for pediatric liquid formulations. MCC pellets were coated *via* spray/fluid bed coating with three aqueous dispersion layers: (I) a drug layer including mainly micronized omeprazole, lactose monohydrate and hypromellose, hydroxypropyl cellulose; (II) a protective layer of hypromellose and (III) an enteric polymer layer with Eudragit® L-30 D-55, 1 N sodium hydroxide and talc. A randomized full factorial design 2^2 + 1 center point optimized the process, focusing on the weight increases of the protective and enteric coatings. Batch 4 was optimal, with 2% second coating and 100% third coating weight increase. Studies included PSD, flow properties, coating uniformity, infrared active pharmaceutical ingredient determination, differential scanning calorimetry, X-ray diffraction, omeprazole content, gastroresistance and dissolution trials. EDS microanalysis confirmed homogeneity. In Batch 4, the omeprazole content was 100%, with 95% gastroresistance and over 80% dissolution in 15 minutes, complying with the established pharmaceutical criteria. Therefore, this formulation could serve as an alternative to existing pediatric formulations that do not provide adequate gastroresistance.

Furthermore, the investigation of Raza et al. [64] explores the formulation of ascorbic acid dual-coated omeprazole pellets to examine their antioxidant effect on omeprazole-induced acute kidney injury (AKI). Eight formulations incorporating Avicel® PH 102, PEG 6000, lactose and Eudragit L-100 in varying ratios were developed using Design of Experiment and extrusion spheronization method, and then analyzed. The optimal formulation, P6, dual-coated with Eudragit L-100 (5% w/v) and ascorbic acid (2% w/v) achieved 98,67% drug loading, 96,54% encapsulation efficiency and 93,45% drug release. IR spectra confirmed drug loading and coating, while X-ray diffraction showed a crystalline nature, and thermal studies indicated enhanced stability. Cytotoxicity analysis verified non-toxicity (97% cell viability). *In vitro* drug release studies demonstrated <20% release in acidic conditions and 99,54% in intestine-like conditions. Elevated uric acid and creatinine levels in mice treated with pure omeprazole, along with histopathological analysis of their kidneys, indicated AKI, in contrast to the groups treated with the formulated pellets. Molecular docking conducted highlighted the potential of combining the above active pharmaceutical ingredients. Hence, the formulation has potent to prevent a serious adverse effect of omeprazole.

2.5.2 Microsphere formulations

Another approach [65] describes the formulation of omeprazole microspheres using the solvent evaporation method. Five distinct formulations were prepared consisting of omeprazole magnesium, HPMC and PVA, among other excipients, in different ratios and then evaluated for their size, surface morphology, percentage yield, drug content, entrapment efficiency and *in vitro* drug release. Formulation number 2 (F2) containing 20%HPMC,1,5% polyvinyl pyrrolidine, 1,5% ethyl cellulose, 2% polyvinyl alcohol and 1,5% hydroxy ethyl cellulose was the optimal formulation showing the highest rates of up to 93,64% drug loading, 92,16% percentage yield, 28,5% drug content, 76,6% entrapment efficiency and 93,64% drug release. Furthermore, the drug release percentages of F2 were 71,3% at 30 minutes and 80,2% at 7 hours—indicating a gradual and continuous release of the drug over time. This formulation offers a sustained type of release, providing a consistent therapeutic effect.

2.5.3 Salts and co-crystals

In the field of salts and co-crystals, two studies were conducted, which combined omeprazole with one nonsteroidal anti-inflammatory drug (NSAID). One of the two studies, by Nascimento et al. [66], described the formulation and characterization of an indomethacin (IND) and omeprazole (OME) salt, as well as an IND:OME co-amorphous system, using liquid assisted grinding with ethanol and dry grinding, respectively. The aim was to reduce IND gastrointestinal side effects due to the presence and action of OME. The IND:OME salt was confirmed *via* Fourier-transform infrared spectroscopy and thermal analysis, showing reduced thermal stability with a melting point of 122.6°C. The co-amorphous system exhibited a single glass transition temperature (Tg) at 51.8°C, indicating homogeneity. Both formulations displayed superior physical stability, with the co-amorphous system maintaining stability for over 100 days. Dissolution studies revealed enhanced rates for both, with the co-amorphous system showing the highest dissolution efficiency (90%). *In vivo* studies in mice demonstrated improved anti-inflammatory and gastroprotective effects, with the IND:OME salt reducing inflammation by 45% and the co-amorphous system by 60%. These results suggest that these formulations have potential

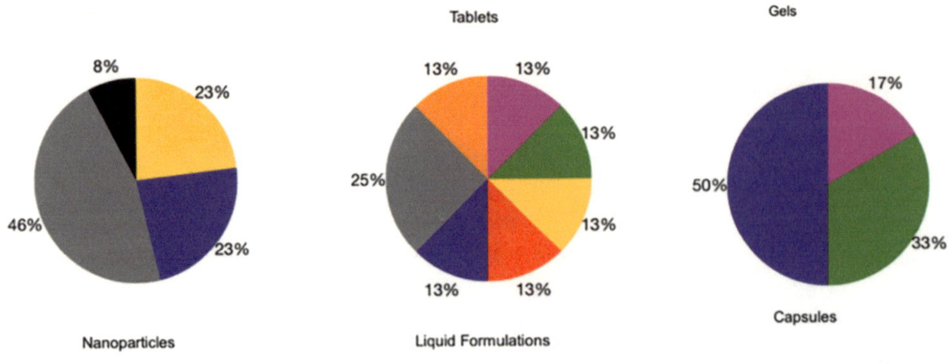

Figure 3.
Type of release of the five most frequent formulation types.

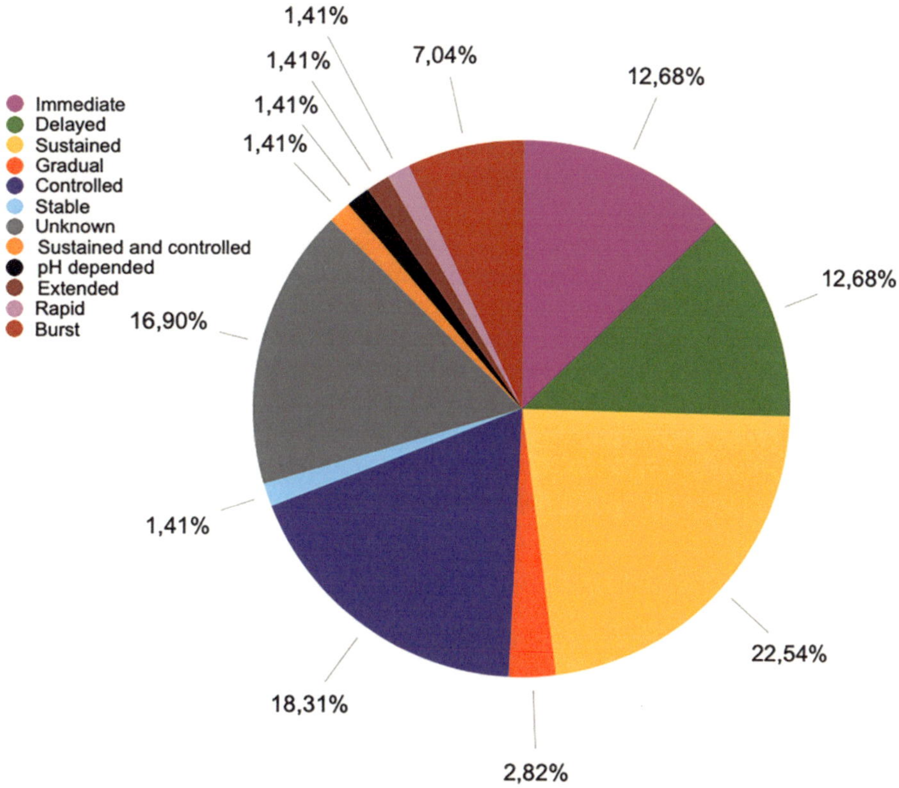

Figure 4.
Frequency of release types of 71 out of 72 formulations. One formulation (semi-solid printable formulation) did not involve a release study in acidic media and therefore was not measured.

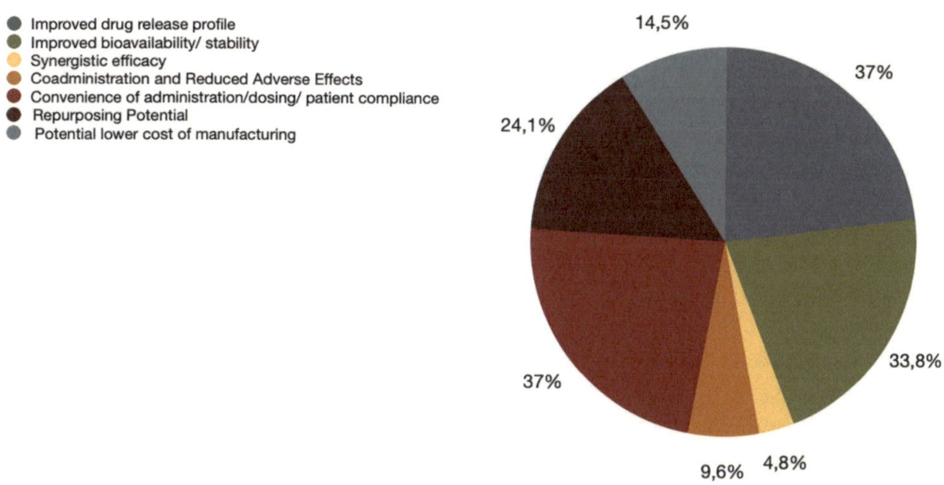

Figure 5.
Revised percentages of each added value.

therapeutic advantages, especially the co-amorphous system, which showed the most significant benefits.

Similarly, the study by de Almeida et al. [67] explored the co-amorphization of Nimesulide (NMS) with six active pharmaceutical ingredients: bicalutamide, isoniazid, metoclopramide, *p*-aminobenzoic acid, piracetam and omeprazole (OME). The aim of the NMS-OME system was to reduce NMS gastrointestinal side effects by the presence and action of OME.

Co-amorphous systems were prepared *via* mechanochemistry and quench cooling. For the NMS-OME system, mechanochemical methods were employed due to OMP's degradation upon melting. Thermal analysis confirmed successful co-amorphization, with NMS-OME cryomilled samples displaying glass transition at 26°C and remaining amorphous for at least 120 days. The cryomilled NMS-OME system demonstrated greater stability compared to cold NG, attributed to cooling below the glass transition temperature, which prevented recrystallization. These findings highlight the potential of cryomilling for stable NMS-OME co-amorphous formulations and their ability to enhance therapeutic outcomes by combining anti-inflammatory and gastroprotective effects (**Figures 3–5**).

3. Discussion

The results presented herein suggest that the dominant and most frequent release types of omeprazole are: "sustained" with a frequency of 22,54%, followed by "controlled" with a frequency of 18,31%. There is also one formulation with a release type named "sustained and controlled" and another one characterized as "pH dependent", which could also belong to the "controlled" type.

Formulations of the sustained release type are fabricated to maintain omeprazole plasma concentrations within a therapeutic window over an extended period of time, thereby prolonging the drug's pharmacological activity. This extended duration of action allows a less frequent dosing plan, which can enhance patient compliance, especially in long-term treatment protocols, such as peptic ulcer disease and gastroesophageal reflux disease management.

Furthermore, controlled-release formulations offer a more precise approach to drug delivery by modulating the release kinetics of omeprazole. These systems ensure a consistent rate of omeprazole release or provide targeted drug delivery, typically to the small intestine, where omeprazole is optimally absorbed. Controlled release mechanisms are particularly beneficial in maintaining steady-state plasma concentrations, thus reducing inter-dose fluctuations that could contribute to suboptimal efficacy or adverse drug reactions [68].

The sustained release type reduces the frequency of dosing and thereby decreasing the risk of missed ones and improving therapeutic outcomes in the management of chronic conditions. Additionally, by minimizing variations in plasma drug levels, controlled-release formulations can enhance omeprazole therapeutic index, improving both safety and efficacy profiles.

In agreement with these findings, the revised percentages of each added value are as follows: In first place, we find the categories "Convenience of administration/dosing/patient compliance" and "Improved drug release profile," both at 37%. Following closely, in the second place is the category "Improved bioavailability/stability" at 33,8%. The "Repurposing Potential" category follows with 24,1%.

This order highlights the main factors driving pharmaceutical innovation today, emphasizing the importance of drug formulations that improve patient adherence and effectiveness in treatment.

The focus on improved bioavailability and stability may indicate a strong need for drugs that are easily absorbed and have longer shelf lives, which can lead to better patient outcomes. Furthermore, the interest in repurposing existing drugs could suggest an aim to optimize them for new therapeutic uses and address unmet medical needs, with accelerated and lower-cost development.

4. OME safety profile-preclinical and clinical considerations

Omeprazole generally has a low rate of adverse effects, primarily involving gastrointestinal symptoms like nausea, abdominal discomfort and altered bowel habits like diarrhea or constipation. Headache is also occasionally reported. Less frequent side effects include dizziness, fatigue, joint pain and skin reactions [69, 70]. As omeprazole is metabolized by CYP2C19 and CYP3A4 enzymes, it can interact with drugs metabolized by these pathways, such as clarithromycin, rifampicin or clopidogrel and others [71]. Omeprazole's suppression of gastric acid may lead to vitamin B12 malabsorption [72]. Furthermore, in patients with additional risk factors, long-term omeprazole treatment raises concerns about osteoporosis [73]. Hypomagnesemia is another reported side effect but the exact mechanism of the Mg^{2+} malabsorption is still unknown [74].

Preclinical studies on omeprazole primarily focus on its pharmacological properties, mechanisms of action, toxicity and safety profile, laying the foundation for clinical trials. Studies like those by Fellenius et al. [75] examined omeprazole's mechanism of action by inhibition of the proton pump in the stomach, demonstrating dose-dependent gastric acid suppression. In addition, research by J. M. Birkett et al. [76] and Meyer et al. [77] outlined omeprazole's pharmacokinetics, showing rapid absorption, metabolism *via* cytochrome P450 system (particularly CYP2C19) and renal excretion, which highlighted the potential for drug-drug interactions. Further studies, such as the study by Blandizzi et al. [78] demonstrated omeprazole's efficacy in healing gastric ulcers and enhancing mucosal protection. Moreover, omeprazole toxicity studies by Ekman et al. [79] and Carlsson et al. [80] showed low acute toxicity in animal studies, with reversible gastric changes and no fetal toxicity or mutagenicity, supporting a favorable safety profile.

These early studies were crucial in advancing omeprazole for clinical use in treating acid-related disorders. Many clinical trials and real-world data studies throughout the years show that omeprazole demonstrates significant efficacy in managing various gastric acid-related disorders. Some examples include a randomized trial about *H. pylori* eradication with omeprazole [81], which showed that the combination of omeprazole with antibiotics (clarithromycin and amoxicillin) was more effective in eradicating *H. pylori* compared to other drug regimens. Additionally, the LOTUS trial (Long-Term Omeprazole Use Study) highlighted omeprazole's ability to reduce symptoms and heal esophagitis in GERD, outperforming placebo and other acid-suppressing drugs like ranitidine [82]. More recently, a real-world study [83] evaluated the effectiveness of omeprazole in treating Acid Peptic Disease. Patients showed significant improvement in symptoms and characterized their therapy as effective, convenient and satisfactory.

Several omeprazole formulations have been withdrawn or discontinued in some markets due to competition, manufacturing challenges, stability issues or safety concerns. For instance, high-dose omeprazole formulations (like Prilosec® 40 mg) were withdrawn due to regulatory concerns over the risks associated with the long-term use of high-dose PPIs. The introduction of alternative PPIs, such as esomeprazole and pantoprazole, also led to the discontinuation of some omeprazole combination therapies and branded versions.

Products like Losec MUPS® (AstraZeneca®) and Zegerid® (Santarus®)—a formulation of omeprazole with sodium bicarbonate—were withdrawn due to inconsistent dissolution rates and stability issues, which affected drug release and effectiveness. Prilosec® suspension had reconstitution stability issues, while intravenous formulations like Rapinex® (Ferring Pharmaceuticals®) were phased out due to storage and stability challenges.

Additionally, contamination and sterility problems in oral formulations (e.g., by Ranbaxy®, Dr. Reddy's® and Teva®) and IV formulations (e.g., by Sandoz® and Hospira®) led to recalls due to quality control failures.

These cases highlight the importance of strict manufacturing practices and strong regulatory oversight, especially for products requiring precise stability, sterility and long-term safety.

5. Conclusions

This chapter aims to present the recent advances in omeprazole's pharmaceutical formulations involving excipients of diverse physicochemical properties. Moreover, its release kinetics from solid, liquid, semi-solid and nanoformulations are described. The improved bioavailability and increased therapeutic efficiency were accompanied by minimal side effects, leading to enhanced patient compliance. The targeted drug delivery and the potential of combination therapy appeared as the added value of nanoformulations over the solid and liquid dosage forms. On the other hand, tablets and other solid dosage forms have already appeared on the market exhibiting patients' friendly dosage forms. To improve the stability, release profile and therapeutic efficacy of omeprazole, a few new formulations have been investigated. Additionally, efforts have been undertaken recently to investigate the full potential of omeprazole and its possible repurposing for other therapeutic uses, including the treatment of cancer. These advancements demonstrate the drug's enduring significance in pharmaceutical innovation as well as its long-standing usefulness in the field of gastroenterology. In the field of cancer treatment, in the context of the repurposing of omeprazole, the nanoformulations have opened new avenues, such as antineoplastic nanomedicines with high therapeutic index.

Conflict of interest

The authors declare no conflict of interest.

Notes/thanks/other declarations

No declarations.

Author details

Ioanna Papoutsi[1,2], Angeliki Siamidi[1], Nefeli Lagopati[3], Maria Gazouli[3], Marilena Vlachou[1*] and Natassa Pippa[1*]

1 Section of Pharmaceutical Technology, Department of Pharmacy, School of Health Sciences, National and Kapodistrian University of Athens, Athens, Greece

2 3rd Department of Internal Medicine, 'Sotiria' Hospital, Athens, Greece

3 Laboratory of Biology, Department of Basic Medical Sciences, Medical School, National and Kapodistrian University of Athens, Athens, Greece

*Address all correspondence to: vlachou@pharm.uoa.gr and natpippa@pharm.uoa.gr

References

[1] Nehra AK, Alexander JA, Loftus CG, Nehra V. Proton pump inhibitors: Review of emerging concerns. Mayo Clinic Proceedings. 2018;**93**:240-246

[2] Shin JM, Munson K, Vagin O, Sachs G. The gastric HK-ATPase: Structure, function, and inhibition. Pflügers Archiv European Journal of Physiology. 2009;**457**:609-622

[3] Welage LS. Pharmacologic properties of proton pump inhibitors. Pharmacotherapy. 2003;**23**:74-80

[4] Wilde MI, McTavish D. Omeprazole, an update of its pharmacology and therapeutic use in acid-related disorders. Drugs. 1994;**48**:91-132. DOI:10.2165/00003495-199448010-00008

[5] Iuga C, Bojita M. Stability study of omeprazole. Farmácia. 2010;**58**(2):203-210

[6] Bozdag SİBEL, Calis SEMA, Sumnu M. Formulation and stability evaluation of enteric-coated omeprazole formulations. STP Pharma Sciences. 1999;**9**(4):321-327

[7] Burnett JE, Balkin ER. Stability and viscosity of a flavored omeprazole oral suspension for pediatric use. American Journal of Health-System Pharmacy. 2006;**63**(22):2240-2247. DOI: 10.2146/ajhp060026

[8] Conley JG, Wolcott RC, Wong E. AstraZeneca, Prilosec, and Nexium: Marketing challenges in the launch of a second-generation drug. Kellogg School of Management Cases. 2017;**1**(1):1-20. DOI: 10.1108/case.kellogg.2016.000028

[9] Srebro J, Brniak W, Mendyk A. Formulation of dosage forms with proton pump inhibitors: State of the art, challenges and future perspectives. Pharmaceutics. 2022;**14**:2043. DOI: 10.3390/pharmaceutics14102043

[10] Spugnini EP, Fais S. Drug repurposing for anticancer therapies. A lesson from proton pump inhibitors. Expert Opinion on Therapeutic Patents. 2019;**30**(1):15-25. DOI: 10.1080/13543776.2020.1704733

[11] Mohapatra SK, Sahoo RN, Mallick S, Mohapatra R. Enteric dissolution enhancement of engineered gastro resistant omeprazole tablets using hydroxypropyl methylcellulose acetate succinate. Indian Journal of Pharmaceutical Education and Research. 2021;**55**(3):677-684. DOI: 10.5530/ijper.55.3.139

[12] Venkata Gopaiah K, Dr PV, Rao D, Narasimha G, Soni LB, Ranjitha CH, et al. Formulation & evaluation omeprazole delayed release tablets. World Journal of Pharmaceutical Research. 2020;**9**(6):2441-2459

[13] Trimukhe A, Rojekar S, Pradeep R, Vavia RR. Deshmukh pulsed plasma surface modified omeprazole microparticles for delayed release application. Journal of Drug Delivery Science and Technology. 2021;**66**:102905. DOI: 10.1016j.jddst.2021.102905. ISSN 1773-2247

[14] Narkhede PS, Singh N, Jain NK. Formulation and characterization of immediate release solid dosage forms of omeprazole. Journal of Pharmaceutical Negative Results. 2022;**13**(10):4879-4883

[15] Kumar G, Jain V, Shende S, Jain P. Formulation and evaluation of bilayer tablets of clarithromycin and omeprazole

against helicobacter pylori infection. The Pharma Innovation Journal. 2019;**8**(1):407-412

[16] Gandrathi Srujana B, Rao CS, Vidhya B, Swapna A, Vivek PV, Chandra DV, et al. Formulation and evaluation of oral disintegrating tablet omeprazole. European Journal of Molecular & Clinical Medicine. 2023;**10**(06):327. ISSN 2515-8260

[17] Bhamare DD, Maru AD, Kothawade PD, Malunjkar DD, Kalpesh S. More formulation and evaluation of fast disintegrating omeprazole tablet by direct compression method. European Journal of Biomedical and Pharmaceutical Sciences. 2023;**10**(12):120-126

[18] Undru Purnima TKV, Rao K, Khiani R. Formulation development and evaluation of omeprazole buccal tablets. International Journal of Research in Pharmacology & Pharmacotherapeutics. 2023;**12**(3):185-196

[19] Kaushal S, Dev D, Prasad DN, Sharma R. Formulation and optimization of omeprazole floating tablet by wet granulation technique. Journal of Drug Delivery and Therapeutics. 2019;**9**(3-s):679-687

[20] Kokate SM, Deokule HA, Desai HR, Vachane Patil RR, Aher SJ, Mule VS, et al. Formulation and evaluation of a tablet by using the solvent evaporation method & solid dispersion method to increase the solubility of omeprazole magnesium. Romanian Journal of Diabetes Nutrition and Metabolic Diseases. 2023;**30**(4):1082-1092. DOI: 10.46389/rjd-2023-1082

[21] Olorunsola EO, Udoh IE, Majekodunmi SO, Odiong IJ, Ebong UO. Inhibition of gastric degradation of omeprazole using a ph-sensitive polymer as a binder in tablet formulation. International Journal of Applied Pharmaceutics. 2021;**13**(5):331-335

[22] Olorunsola EO, Adedokun MO, Olisakwe PC, Mfonobong F. Alozie *in vitro* evaluation of prosopis gum matrix for duodenum-targeted delivery of omeprazole. Journal of Applied Pharmaceutical Science. 2022;**12**(06):164-171

[23] Bikiaris ND, Christodoulou E, Bikiaris R, Barmpalexis P, Kostoglou M, Tsamesidis I, et al. Fabrication of chitosan-based omeprazole matrix tablets. In: *In Vitro* Modified Release Studies. Journal of Applied Pharmacy (Brussels: Longdom Publishing). 2024;**16**(5):1000440. ISSN: 1920-4159

[24] Agapakis G, Siamidi A, Kikionis S, Vlachou M, Pippa N. A thermal-analysis-technique-based mechanistic approach toward the release of omeprazole from solid dosage forms. Scientia Pharmaceutica. 2024;**92**:8. DOI: 10.3390/scipharm92010008

[25] Parihar A, Prajapati BG, Patel K, Paliwal H. Formulation, evaluation, and optimization of the omeprazole magnesium multi-unit particulate controlled release tablets using different concentrations of polymers. IP International Journal of Comprehensive and Advanced Pharmacology. 2023;**7**(4):211-217. DOI: 10.18231/j.ijcaap.2022.040

[26] Juère E, Del Favero G, Masse F, Marko D, Popat A, Florek J, et al. Gastro-protective protein-silica nanoparticles formulation for oral drug delivery: *In vitro* release, cytotoxicity and mitochondrial activity. European Journal of Pharmaceutics and Biopharmaceutics. 2020;**151**:171-180. DOI: 10.1016/j.ejpb.2020.03.015. Epub 2020 Apr 14

[27] Patel D, Yadav S, Sharma P, Tyagi N, Katiyar PK. Formulation and evaluation of omeprazole nanoparticles for Gred African. Journal of Biological Sciences. 2024;**6**(Si3):2988-2999. DOI: 10.48047AFJBS.6.Si3.2024.2988-2999

[28] Chandra SM, Dharan SS, Ajikumar A. Formulation and evaluation of gastroretentive floating microballoons containing selected anti-ulcer drug. Journal of Pharmaceutical Sciences and Research. 2021;**13**(1):49-63

[29] Afonso Urich JA, Fedorko A, Hölzer B, Khinast J. Evidence of reliable gastro-resistance of novel enteric ready-to-fill capsules simplifying pharmaceutical manufacturing. Pharmaceutics. 2023;**15**(11):2592. DOI: 10.3390/pharmaceutics15112592

[30] Kumisbek G, Vetchý D, Kadyrbay A. Development of a new bioequivalent omeprazole product. Medicina (Kaunas, Lithuania). 2024;**60**(3):427. DOI: 10.3390/medicina60030427

[31] Geng L, Han L, Huang L, Wu Z, Wu Z, Qi X. High anti-acid omeprazole lightweight capsule for gastro-enteric system acid-related disorders treatment. Journal of Clinical Gastroenterology and Treatment. 2019;**5**(2). DOI: 10.23937/2469-584X/1510068

[32] Huang GQ, Zhang ZK, Cheng LY, Xiao JX. Intestine-targeted delivery potency of O carboxymethyl chitosan-coated layer-by-layer microcapsules: An *in vitro* and *in vivo* evaluation. Materials Science & Engineering. C, Materials for Biological Applications. 2019;**105**:110129. DOI: 10.1016/j.msec.2019.110129. Epub 2019 Aug 24

[33] Sanni G, Santosh K. Formulation and evaluation of combined dosage form of diclofenac sodium (mini tablet) and omeprazole sodium in capsule devices. Journal of Pharmaceutical Research Science & Technology. 2022;**6**(1):162. DOI: 10.31531/jprst.1000162

[34] Kim WK, Cho HH, Lee GW, et al. Alleviated side effects and improved efficiency of omeprazole using oral thin film: *In vitro* evaluation. Macromolecular Research. 2019;**28**:417-424. DOI: 10.1007/s13233-020-8060-x

[35] Rouaz-El Hajoui K, Herrada-Manchón H, Rodríguez-González D, Fernández MA, Aguilar E, Suñé-Pou M, et al. Pellets and gummies: Seeking a 3D printed gastro-resistant omeprazole dosage for paediatric administration. International Journal of Pharmaceutics. 2023;**643**:123289. DOI: 10.1016/j.ijpharm.2023.123289. Epub 2023 Aug 2

[36] Soni A, Kataria MK. Formulation and evaluation of floating *in situ* gel of omeprazole magnesium for oral drug delivery system. Asian Journal of Pharmaceutical and Clinical Research. 2021;**14**(9):44-52. DOI: 10.22159/ajpcr.2021.v14i9.42231

[37] Heikal EJ, Kaoud RM, Gad S, Mokhtar HI, Aldahish AA, Alzlaiq WA, et al. Design and optimization of omeprazole-curcumin-loaded hydrogel beads coated with chitosan for treating peptic ulcers. Pharmaceuticals (Basel). 2023;**16**(6):795. DOI: 10.3390/ph16060795

[38] Balakrishnan B, Sarojini BK, Kodoth AK, Dayananda BS, Venkatesha R. Fabrication and characterization of tamarind seed gum based novel hydrogel for the targeted delivery of omeprazole magnesium. International Journal of Biological Macromolecules. 2024;**258**(Pt 1):128758. DOI: 10.1016/j.ijbiomac.2023.128758. Epub 2023 Dec 15

[39] Ullah I, Alhodaib A, Naz I, Ahmad W, Ullah H, Amin A, et al. Fabrication of novel omeprazole-based chitosan coated Nanoemulgel formulation for potential anti-microbia; *in vitro* and *ex vivo* characterizations. Polymers. 2023;**15**(5):1298. DOI: 10.3390/polym15051298

[40] Jingrong M, Du Chaoqun ZY, Jing Z, Yafang L, Mingwei Z. Important application value of injectable hydrogels loaded with omeprazole Schiff base complex in the treatment of pancreatitis. Open Chemistry. 2023;**21**(1):20230147. DOI: 10.1515/chem-2023-0147

[41] Kathiravan G. Formulation of novel nano transdermal using effective combination of acyclovir and omeprazole for enhanced anti-viral activity. International Journal of Pharmaceutical research and Applications. 2024;**9**(6):80-97

[42] Chachlioutaki K, Iordanopoulou A, Bouropoulos N, Meikopoulos T, Gika H, Ritzoulis C, et al. Pediatric and geriatric-friendly buccal foams: Enhancing omeprazole delivery for patients encountering swallowing difficulties. Journal of Pharmaceutical Sciences. 2023;**112**(10):2644-2654. DOI: 10.1016/j.xphs.2023.07.025. Epub 2023 Aug 6

[43] Bestebreurtje P, Roeleveld N, Knibbe CAJ, van Sorge AA, Plötz FB, de Wildt SN. Development and stability study of an omeprazole suppository for infants. European Journal of Drug Metabolism and Pharmacokinetics. 2020;**45**(5):627-633. DOI: 10.1007/s13318-020-00629-1

[44] Khatibi A, Zahedi P, Ghourchian H, Lari AS. Development of microfluidic-based cellulose acetate phthalate nanoparticles containing omeprazole for antiulcer activity: *In vitro* and *in vivo* evaluations. European Polymer Journal. 2021;**147**(1):110294. DOI: 10.1016 j.eurpolymj.2021.110294

[45] Rezazadeh M, Safaran R, Minaiyan M, Mostafavi A. Preparation and characterization of Eudragit L 100-55/chitosan enteric nanoparticles containing omeprazole using general factorial design: *In vitro/in vivo* study. Research in Pharmaceutical Sciences. 2021;**16**(4):358-369. DOI: 10.4103/1735-5362.319574

[46] Li L, Jing J, Yang S, Fang S, Liu W, Wang C, et al. *Bletilla striata* polysaccharide nanoparticles improved the therapeutic efficacy of omeprazole on the rat gastric ulcer induced by ethanol. Molecular Pharmaceutics. 2023;**20**(4):1996-2008. DOI: 10.1021/acs.molpharmaceut.2c00922. Epub 2023 Feb 24

[47] Manivannan S, Sivaraman H, Murugesan R, et al. Omeprazole and H2S releasing agents encapsulated in chitosan nanoparticles to enhance healing process against indomethacin-induced gastric ulcer model. Journal of Materials Research. 2023;**38**:3089-3109. DOI: 10.1557s43578-023-01030-9

[48] Moretto S, Santos Silva A, Diaz de Tuesta JL, Roman FF, Cortesi R, Bertão AR, et al. Comprehensive characterization and development of multi-core shell superparamagnetic nanoparticles for controlled delivery of drugs and their kinetic release modelling. Materials Today Chemistry. 2023;**33**:101748. DOI: 10.1016/j.mtchem.2023.101748. ISSN 2468-5194

[49] Sun L, Liu Y, Liu X, Wang R, Gong J, Saferali A, et al. Nano-enabled reposition of proton pump inhibitors for TLR inhibition: Toward a new targeted nanotherapy for acute lung injury. Advanced Science (Weinh).

2022;**9**(3):e2104051. DOI: 10.1002/advs.202104051. Epub 2021 Nov 23

[50] Eswar K, Sankaranarayanan SA, Srivastava R, Harijan D, Prabusankar G, Rengan AK. Omeprazole-loaded copper nanoparticles for mitochondrial damage mediated synergistic anticancer activity against melanoma cells. ACS Applied Bio Materials. 2024;7(7):4795-4803. DOI: 10.1021/acsabm.4c0063

[51] Wang T, Xiao G, Lu Q, Zhou Y, Wang S, Liang X, et al. Synergistic lysosomal impairment and ER stress activation for boosted autophagy dysfunction based on Te double-headed nano-bullets. Small. 2022;**18**(27):e2201585. DOI: 10.1002/smll.202201585. Epub 2022 May 29

[52] Sharifzadeh B, Mahmoodi NO, Ravanan A. Synthesis of omeprazole@AgNPs and omeprazole sulfide@AgNPs and considering their antibacterial properties. 2023;**1**. DOI: 10.20944/preprints202309.1246.v1 [Preprints]

[53] Ravanan A, Mahmoodi O, N., Sharifzadeh, B., Majlesi, F. Green synthesis of omeprazole@AgNPs, omeprazole sulfide@AgNPs, pantoprazole@AgNPs and pantoprazole sulfide@AgNPs by using leaf extract of Ruta, Pimpinella saxifrage and mango. International Journal of New Chemistry. 2023;**11**(1):70-81. DOI: 10.22034/ijnc.2023.2011981.1359

[54] Zia A, Shahzad A, Riaz N, Khan S, Farooq U, Bukhari SM, et al. Enhancement efficacy of omeprazole by conjugation with silver nanoparticles as a urease inhibitor. Green Processing and Synthesis. 2024;**13**(1). DOI: 10.1515/gps-2023-0229

[55] Mobarak Qamsari E, Kermanshahi RK, Erfan M, Ghadam P. Microencapsulation of omeprazole by *Lactobacillus acidophilus* ATCC 4356 surface layer protein and evaluation of its stability in acidic condition. Iranian Journal of Pharmaceutical Sciences. 2020;**19**(4):240-254. DOI: 10.22037/ijpr.2019.111681.13306

[56] Ronchi F, Sereno A, Paide M, Sacré P, Guillaume G, Stéphenne V, et al. Development and evaluation of an omeprazole-based delayed-release liquid oral dosage form. International Journal of Pharmaceutics. 2019;**567**:118416. DOI: 10.1016/j.ijpharm.2019.06.007. Epub 2019 Jun 5

[57] Boscolo O, Perra F, Salvo L, Buontempo F, Lucangioli S. Formulation and stability study of omeprazole oral liquid suspension for pediatric patients. Hospital Pharmacy. 2020;**55**(5):314-322. DOI: 10.1177/0018578719844704. Epub 2019 Apr 25

[58] Denga W, Wanga Z, Zhanga Y, Chena Q, Xiaoa X, Redshawb C. Study on the preparation technology of omeprazole vesicles. Russian Journal of General Chemistry. 2021;**91**(11):2311-2319. ISSN 1070-3632

[59] Gupta MK, Sreedharan SK, Sajeeth CI. Design development and characterization of omeprazole loaded nanosuspension. Journal of Pharmaceutical Negative Results. 2022;**13**(Special Issue 8):1195-1208

[60] Diefenthaeler HS, Bianchin MD, Marques MS, Nonnenmacher JL, Bender ET, Bender JG, et al. Omeprazole nanoparticles suspension: Development of a stable liquid formulation with a view to pediatric administration. International Journal of Pharmaceutics. 2020;**589**:119818. DOI: 10.1016j.ijpharm.2020.119818. Epub 2020 Aug 29

[61] Sanad MH, Eyssa HM, Marzook FA, et al. Preparation and bioevaluation

of [99mTc]tricarbonyl omeprazole for gastric ulcer localization in mice. Radiochemistry. 2022;**64**:54-61. DOI: 10.1134/S106636222201009X

[62] Anusha M, Bhagawati ST, Manjunath K. Formulation and evaluation of floating pellets of omeprazole by extrusion spheronization method. Journal of Biomedical and Pharmaceutical Research. 2020;**9**(2):32-37

[63] Rouaz-El-Hajoui K, García-Montoya E, López-Urbano A, Romero-Obon M, Chiclana-Rodríguez B, Fraschi-Nieto A, et al. Optimisation of the manufacturing process of organic-solvent-free omeprazole enteric pellets for the paediatric population: Full factorial design. Pharmaceutics. 2023;**15**(11):2587. DOI: 10.3390/pharmaceutics15112587

[64] Raza H, Abrar A, Ashraf A, Manzoor S, Shamim R, Siddique F, et al. Design, synthesis, evaluation, and molecular docking study of ascorbic acid dual-coated omeprazole pellets and the antioxidative effect of ascorbic acid on omeprazole-induced renal injury in an animal model. ACS Omega. 2023;**9**(1):1143-1155. DOI: 10.1021/acsomega.3c07396

[65] Balmiki R, Patel S, Chadar C, Jain R, Vishwakarma H, Dangi Y, et al. Preparation and optimization of mucoadhesive microsphere of omeprazole in the treatment of peptic ulcer. International Journal of Pharmaceutics and Drug Research. 2023;**12**:228-239

[66] Nascimento ALCS, Martins ICB, Spósito L, Morais-Silva G, Duarte JL, Rades T, et al. Indomethacin-omeprazole as therapeutic hybrids? Salt and co-amorphous systems enhancing physicochemical and pharmacological properties. International Journal of Pharmaceutics. 2024;**653**:123857. DOI: 10.1016/j.ijpharm.2024.123857. Epub 2024 Jan 26

[67] de Almeida AC, Ferreira PO, Porto MV, et al. Novel nimesulide multicomponent solid forms: Screening, synthesis, thermoanalytical study and characterization. Journal of Thermal Analysis and Calorimetry. 2024. DOI: 10.1007/s10973-024-13189-2

[68] Lee VH, Robinson JR. Sustained and Controlled Release Drug Delivery System. New York: Marcel Dekker; 1978. pp. 71-121, 138-171

[69] Richter JE, Kahrilas PJ, Johanson J, Maton P, Breiter JR, Hwang C, et al. Efficacy and safety of esomeprazole compared with omeprazole in GERD patients with erosive esophagitis: A randomized controlled trial. The American Journal of Gastroenterology. 2001;**96**(3):656-665. DOI: 10.1111/j.1572-0241.2001.3600_b.x

[70] Sölvell L. The clinical safety of omeprazole. Digestion. 1990;**47**(Suppl. 1):59-63. DOI: 10.1159/000200519. discussion 76

[71] Ben Ghezala I, Luu M, Bardou M. An update on drug-drug interactions associated with proton pump inhibitors. Expert Opinion on Drug Metabolism & Toxicology. 2022;**18**(5):337-346. DOI: 10.1080/17425255.2022.2098107. Epub 2022 Jul 11

[72] Choudhury A, Jena A, Jearth V, Dutta AK, Makharia G, Dutta U, et al. Vitamin B12 deficiency and use of proton pump inhibitors: A systematic review and meta-analysis. Expert Review of Gastroenterology & Hepatology. 2023;**17**(5):479-487. DOI: 10.1080/17474124.2023.2204229. Epub 2023 Apr 19

[73] Lespessailles E, Toumi H. Proton pump inhibitors and bone health: An update narrative review. International Journal of Molecular Sciences. 2022;**23**(18):10733. DOI: 10.3390/ijms231810733

[74] Gommers LMM, Hoenderop JGJ, de Baaij JHF. Mechanisms of proton pump inhibitor-induced hypomagnesemia. Acta Physiologica (Oxford, England). 2022;**235**(4):e13846. DOI: 10.1111/apha.13846. Epub 2022 Jun 14

[75] Fellenius E, Berglindh T, Sachs G, Olbe L, Elander B, Sjöstrand SE, et al. Substituted benzimidazoles inhibit gastric acid secretion by blocking (H^{++} K^{+})ATPase. Nature. 1981;**290**(5802):159-161. DOI: 10.1038/290159a0

[76] Birkett DJ, Andersson T, Miners JO. Assays of omeprazole metabolism as a substrate probe for human CYP isoforms. Methods in Enzymology. 1996;**272**:132-139. DOI: 10.1016/s0076-6879(96)72016-5

[77] Meyer UA. Interaction of proton pump inhibitors with cytochromes P450: Consequences for drug interactions. The Yale Journal of Biology and Medicine. 1996;**69**(3):203-209

[78] Blandizzi C, Gherardi G, Marveggio C, Natale G, Carignani D, Del Tacca M. Mechanisms of protection by omeprazole against experimental gastric mucosal damage in rats. Digestion. 1995;**56**(3):220-229. DOI: 10.1159/000201247

[79] Ekman L, Hansson E, Havu N, Carlsson E, Lundberg C. Toxicological studies on omeprazole. Scandinavian Journal of Gastroenterology. Supplement. 1985;**108**:53-69

[80] Carlsson E, Larsson H, Mattsson H, Ryberg B, Sundell G. Pharmacology and toxicology of omeprazole—with special reference to the effects on the gastric mucosa. Scandinavian Journal of Gastroenterology. Supplement. 1986;**118**:31-38. DOI: 10.3109/00365528609090884

[81] Pieramico O, Zanetti MV, Innerhofer M, Malfertheiner P. Omeprazole-based dual and triple therapy for the treatment of *Helicobacter pylori* infection in peptic ulcer disease: A randomized trial. Helicobacter. 1997;**2**(2):92-97. DOI: 10.1111/j.1523-5378.1997.tb00065.x

[82] Galmiche J, Hatlebakk J, Attwood S, et al. Laparoscopic antireflux surgery vs esomeprazole treatment for chronic GERD: The LOTUS randomized clinical trial. Journal of the American Medical Association. 2011;**305**(19):1969-1977. DOI: 10.1001/jama.2011.626

[83] Jain S, Shamrao Kulkarni S, Mahapatra JR, Todi D, Petare AU, Banerjee R, et al. Effectiveness of omeprazole in acid peptic disease: A real-world, patient-reported outcome measures study. Cureus. 2023;**15**(7):e41994. DOI: 10.7759/cureus.41994